TIME DISTORTION
IN
HYPNOSIS

TIME DISTORTION IN HYPNOSIS

An Experimental and Clinical Investigation

Second Edition

By Linn F. Cooper, M.D.

and

Milton H. Erickson, M.A., M.D.

CROWN HOUSE PUBLISHING
www.crownhouse.co.uk

Published by
Crown House Publishing Ltd
Crown Buildings
Bancyfelin, Carmarthen, Wales, SA33 5ND, UK
www.crownhouse.co.uk
and
Crown House Publishing Limited
P.O. Box 2223, Williston, VT. 05495
www. CHPUS.com

Reprinted 2002 Crown House Publishing Ltd.
Reprinted with permission of Ardent Media, Inc.
First Ardent Media Edition 1982
Copyright © 1959 by Linn F. Cooper, M.D.

Library of Congress Cataloging in Publication Data

Cooper, Linn F.
  Time distortion in hypnosis.

  Reprint. Originally published: 2nd ed. Baltimore:
Williams & Wilkins, 1959.
  Bibliography: p.
  Includes index.
  1. Hypnotism. 2. Time perception disorders.
3. Learning, Psychology of. I. Erickson, Milton H.
II. Title.
RC497.C6   1982   154.7'7   82-6633
ISBN 1-89983-695-0   AACR2

Preface to the Second Edition

The explication, in the first edition of this book, of the experimental and clinical aspects of hypnotic time distortion as a specific concept and a new technique was a most intriguing task for the authors. The reception accorded the book, as evidenced by favorable reviews, the exhaustion of first and second printings, the receipt of letters of inquiry about experimental procedures from research workers in many parts of the country, even from abroad, and the favorable comment from scores of clinicians on their own utilization of hypnotic time distortion, have been most stimulating.

However, the authors can take credit for only a small part of this. The timing of the first edition, 1954, was both fortuitous and fortunate. The impetus given by World War II to the scientific use of hypnosis was continuing in the form of progressive development of general medical interest. The dental profession, long interested, manifested this by taking the lead in employing hypnosis in office practice. The efforts previously made by the psychology departments of various universities to arouse a widespread interest in research in hypnosis took on a new vitality. Contemporaneous with this constantly growing interest, the first edition was issued, and it profited greatly therefrom. Additionally, it was a book written by physicians in which purely experimental and purely clinical work with new and different applications were presented—this at a time of searching for new techniques for special adaptation to the problems of psychosomatic medicine.

Less than a year after the first edition was published, but expressive only of the fact that interest in scientific hypnosis was not limited to any one country, the British Medical Association formally approved of the medical use and teaching of hypnosis and disapproved its use by the laity. Also in 1955, Marquette University School of Dentistry, and in 1956, Tufts University School of Dental Medicine, to give examples of academic interest, conducted formal seminars on hypnosis as a part of postgraduate instruction. Then, in 1957, The American Society of Clinical Hypnosis was organized on a national level with international affiliations with other national scientific societies and with a membership based on a doctoral degree in psychology, dentistry or medicine. Thus, there was inaugurated an era of generalized professional approval of scientific hypnosis and the enlistment of the interest and participation of clinicians everywhere.

In 1958, the American Medical Association formally approved the use and teaching of hypnosis as a medical methodology of significant value. Further recognition was accorded by other national and state or regional medical and dental societies.

Against the background of this interest, a second edition is being issued as a restatement of a methodology offering an opportunity for both research and clinical application in a wide variety of problems in medicine and dentistry, both physiological and psychological. Aside from minor changes and additions to the first section of this book, the justification for calling this issue a second edition is the fact of an addition of a relatively brief but new and different third section, clinically oriented but with a variety of experimental significances. This new section, in the authors' opinion, constitutes a decidedly important elaboration of another significant aspect of hypnotic time distortion—an aspect only briefly mentioned in discussions in the first edition, but which was entirely overlooked for elaboration both experimentally and clinically. This phase of hypnotic time distortion is the shortening or condensation of subjective time experience, the converse of the subjective lengthening or time expansion treated at length in the first edition. Two types of observational findings are employed to explicate the manifestations of subjective time condensation, those deriving from unplanned spontaneous developments and those arising from a systematic employment of time condensation as a clinical measure in the handling of subjectively difficult or distressing experiences.

With this new section added to the book, the authors feel that they have now restated and completed a reasonably comprehensive description of the concept of subjective hypnotic time distortion. It is their hope that the experimental and clinical work of others will continue the task of investigating the psychosomatic problems involved in subjective time values, both expanded and condensed, and which are so important, whether in health or illness, in the experiential life of the individual.

L. F. C.

M. H. E.

Preface to the First Edition

The work reported in this monograph was done, as occasion arose, in the period between February 1948 and May 1954. As the experiments progressed, the findings led to speculation concerning their significance and possible implications. So intriguing were some of the questions raised that, rather than attempting to study exhaustively any single one of them, a number of pilot experiments involving different problems were carried out. In other words it was, in a sense, like making a series of short exploratory trips in various directions into a strange land. It is the hope of the authors that this presentation may stimulate others to venture further.

In Part I the author has freely drawn upon two articles, "Time Distortion in Hypnosis, I" and "Time Distortion in Hypnosis, II", originally published in the *Bulletin of the Georgetown University Medical Center*. Furthermore, Chapters 18, 19, and 22 are here reprinted, with some changes, from articles appearing in the *Journal of Psychology* and in *Science*. On the other hand, a good deal of previously unpublished work is included in Part I. Part II, in which case reports are presented, is entirely new except for one section.

The authors are most grateful to Dr. Harold Rosen for his interest and encouragement during the experimental phase of the work. They also wish to thank the Georgetown University Medical Center, the Macmillan Company, the American Association for the Advancement of Science, and Dr. Carl Murchison for permission to use material formerly published by them.

L. F. C.
M. H. E.

Foreword

This is the only detailed study of a single, specific hypnotic technique —aside from that of symptom-disappearance by direct verbal suggestion—with which I personally am familiar. As such, it constitutes a signal contribution to the field.

Dr. Cooper's first article on *Time Distortion* appeared in 1948. In this, and in his five subsequent publications on the subject, he has very specifically restricted his definition of the term to that of a marked difference between the seeming duration and the clock reading of a given interval of time. This of itself, as we all know, is a not uncommon phenomenon. It may occur during the stress of battle, while dreaming, or when under the influence of drugs like mescalin (peyote). The concept, as developed by Dr. Cooper, however, connotes slowing of the subjective perception of time, under rigidly set and specifically stated conditions, by means of hypnotic techniques which he describes in detail in this book.

A number of criticisms have been levelled against Dr. Cooper's previously published research on the subject. It has been stated, for instance, that he attempts to explain complex psychological processes by semantic devices, that he is extremely naïve psychologically, and that what he believes to be *facilitation of learning* (and what others sometimes term *learning effectiveness*) could well be conditioned by factors other than those implied by time distortion, although what these factors are has not been described.

If, nevertheless, these criticisms be stated, not negatively but positively and constructively, it soon becomes apparent that the whole problem of learning effectiveness—and the factors underlying this—comes to the fore. Conditions have been formulated, both in his earlier publications and in this volume, which may well be taken into consideration in any further experimental study of the learning process. This is a meaningful and significant contribution, and must be considered of prime importance. With marked alteration in time perception, so it seems, accelerated mental activity appears possible. It is this, in fact, which is discussed, investigated and evaluated, from variant philosophical, psychologic and psychiatric angles of approach, throughout this book. One must commend the industry and the diligence with which during the past six years Dr. Cooper has so conscientiously investigated and developed so important a concept.

Time distortion under hypnosis is one form of time manipulation. Its therapeutic implications were detailed by Dr. Erickson, in an article written in collaboration with Dr. Cooper, as early as 1950. The second half of this work, however, lists them in detail—and with significant illustrative case material. Stress is on the adjuvant use of this very specific hypnotic technique in attempts on the part of the therapist to help his patient most rapidly and most meaningfully.

This means, of course, that the experiential background of the patient—his capacities, his behavior, his thinking and his emotions—must all constantly be taken into consideration. Inter-personal, intra-personal and object relationships are therefore brought into sharp focus. The problems involved, and the ingenuity with which they can be solved, may be seen with the sharpness of caricature from the abstracted case protocols incorporated in the second half of this monograph.

Dr. Erickson's previous research with hypnotic techniques has placed him in the forefront of the world's authorities on the subject. He has studied, devised and evaluated a number of hypnotic techniques—and reported his results in some of the most significant of the publications on the subject. Our understanding of the motivational bases of human behavior has been increased by the experimental psychological, and the clinical therapeutic, research which he and his co-workers have published on crystal gazing, automatic writing, the induction of parallel experimental neuroses, the silent consideration of other non-neurotic and more adequate methods of resolving factors underlying symptoms, etc. His work on time regression, which has already been published, and his work on time progression, which is now in publication, is of prime importance. And his present study of possible therapeutic implications, when utilized with specific patients, of time distortion is equally significant.

To summarize: the concept of time distortion, in the very specific sense in which that term is defined in this work, but in its non-therapeutic implications, is discussed, investigated, and evaluated in the first half of this book by Dr. Cooper. In so doing, conditions are formulated which can—and perhaps must—be taken into consideration later on in experimental studies of the learning process. The clinical phenomena involved, with specific reference to therapeutic applications, are discussed and studied by Dr. Erickson, along with meaningful illustrative case material, in the second half of this work.

All of us who work in the field owe a debt of gratitude to the two authors for this detailed contribution of theirs.

It is a privilege and an honor to be invited to write the Foreword to this monograph.

HAROLD ROSEN, PH.D., M.D.
School of Medicine
The Johns Hopkins University
Baltimore, Maryland

Contents

Since the human mind first wakened from slumber, and was allowed to give itself free rein, it has never ceased to feel the profoundly mysterious nature of time-consciousness, of the progression of the world in time,—of Becoming.

—HERMANN WEYL

PART I

Experimental Studies

Linn F. Cooper, M.D.

WASHINGTON, D. C.

CHAPTER 1

Introduction

In essence, the studies here presented concern *experience* induced in the hypnotized subject as a result of verbal suggestion. By experience we mean the contents of the subject's field of awareness. It thus includes all those entities which are immediately known, among which are sensations, drives, feelings, emotions, images, meaning-tone, volition, etc., and memories thereof. It is important to point out that this definition makes no stipulation as to whether a given experiential entity is demonstrable to others or not. A chair that two persons look at and describe to each other is an experiential entity just as is an hallucinated chair known only to one individual. It is well known, of course, that the field of awareness may be altered by the direction of one's attention, but this is not an important consideration here. On the other hand, under the above definition, we cannot recognize such a term as "unconscious experience" when this term means "experience" of which the subject is not aware. An unconscious person may be aware of experience in the form of a dream, of course. Thus he is conscious of the dream, though clinically unconscious. On the other hand, when there is no awareness, there is no experience in the sense in which we shall use the word.

Let us suppose that a man participates in a 15-minute conference but makes no note of the time. After the conference we ask him, "How long did the conference last?" and he replies, "I don't know, I didn't note the time." We then ask him, "How long did its duration *seem* to be?" and his reply is, "It seemed to be about 25 minutes." This statement as to how long the interval between the beginning and end of the conference seemed to be, we shall call the *seeming duration* of the interval.

Let us now suppose that our friend, instead of ignoring the time, noted that it was nine o'clock when he started the conference, and that it was 9:15 when he ended it. It is quite obvious then, provided the clock was running properly, that the tip of the minute-hand moved over 15 one-minute divisions during the interval between the start and the termination of the conference. In this case our friend, if asked how long the

1

conference lasted, can truthfully reply, "15 minutes." In so stating this result of his clock observations, i.e., that the interval was 15 minutes long, he is giving what we shall term the *clock reading* of the interval.

These two concepts, seeming duration and clock reading of an interval, will be discussed at greater length in another section. We wish to point out here, however, that the units employed have the same name in each case (minutes in this instance) and that all intervals that can be known in experience can be considered from both points of view. Furthermore, depending upon circumstances, they may be in close agreement or at wide variance. In the above examples, the two differed by 10 minutes. When there is a *marked* difference between the seeming duration and the clock reading of a given interval, we say that *time distortion* is present.

As will be pointed out later, both duration and sequence are known in immediate experience, for we can say of two events that one is before or after or simultaneous with the other and, within limits, we can readily distinguish between the lengths of two successive intervals. This knowing of sequence and duration is effected by means of our *time sense* or sense of *experiential time,* and the present studies were undertaken in order to learn whether or not the sense of duration of an interval can be deliberately altered by means of verbal suggestion in the trance state. We shall have a good deal to say about experiential time in the following pages, but it is well to note here that it is apparently a concept which is not readily grasped by some individuals. The reason for this is not at present clear, but it has led to a considerable amount of difficulty in the communication of our findings to such persons, who have not infrequently stated that they had not the slightest idea as to what the authors were driving at.

The initial experiments involved the use of a metronome which was striking at a constant rate of one stroke per second. The suggestion was given to the hypnotized subject that the metronome was being gradually slowed down, and the reports indicate that the subject actually experienced a marked slowing in the rhythm. In other words, the seeming duration of the intervals reportedly became greatly prolonged.

The next studies involved the participation by the subject in hallucinatory activity during the seemingly prolonged intervals, and the results indicated that large amounts of such activity could be engaged in under these circumstances. In other words, with the clock reading between metronome strokes one second, and the seeming duration of the intervals one minute, the subject reported, during ten successive strokes, an amount of activity that was appropriate to ten *minutes* rather than ten seconds. It is especially significant that this activity *seemed to progress at a normal or customary rate* as far as the subject was concerned.

Subsequently, a technique was developed whereby hallucinatory activity could be produced under conditions of time distortion without the use of a metronome. The following report of an experiment will serve to give the reader a general idea of the procedure which, with variations, was used in most of this study. The subject, who was in a moderately deep trance, lay motionless on a couch with her *eyes closed* throughout. E. stands for experimenter, S. for subject.

1. E. What would you like to do now?
2. S. I'd like to spend a half hour riding in an automobile.
3. E. Now listen to me carefully. When I give you the starting signal by saying "Now," you're going to spend at least a half hour of your special time riding in an automobile, and it's going to be a nice ride. Here comes the starting signal, "Now."

(Ten *seconds* later)

4. E. Now make your mind a blank.

(The subject was then waked.)

5. E. Tell me what happened, please.
6. S. (The subject told how she and her sister, both children at the time, sat on the back seat of the car and counted cows seen along the way. Her sister won the game, counting 45 to her 42. Then they decided to count licenses bearing the letter "C". This was slow, for there was but little traffic. They both saw the same ones, 14 in all. Then they stopped at a roadside stand to buy lemonade from a little girl with pigtails and several missing teeth because they "felt sorry for her".)
7. E. Was it real?
8. S. Yes.
9. E. Were there any omissions?
10. S. No.
11. E. Did you enjoy it?
12. S. Oh, yes!
13. E. How long did it seem?
14. S. A half hour easy.

It is most important to point out that the subject lay motionless during this hallucinatory experience.

The following terminology is applied to the various parts of the above procedure:

Item 3. This contains an introductory expression, "Now listen to me carefully. When I give you the starting signal by saying 'now'." "You're going to spend at least a half hour of your special time" is the assigning of the *suggested personal time*. The expression "riding in an automobile, and it's going to be a nice ride," is known as the *activity instruction*. "Here comes the starting signal, 'Now'," is self-explanatory.

Item 4. This expression is known as the *termination signal*.

Item 5. This is the request for a report.

Item 6. This is the subject's report.

Item 13. This is a request for the *seeming duration* of the experience.

Item 14. This is the seeming duration as reported by the subject.

The 10-second clock reading of the interval between the starting signal and the termination signal constitutes the *allotted time*. The interval itself, during which the subject engages in the suggested activity, is the *activity interval*.

COMMENTS

It is evident from Items 1 and 2 that in this particular experiment the subject was given a choice of activities. This is by no means necessary, but is of some importance during training.

The fact that the seeming duration (Item 14) of the activity was "a half hour easy", whereas the clock reading was 10 seconds, indicated that *time distortion* was present.

The subject's report in Item 6 is allegedly a simple narrative account of a trip she took in an automobile, and might just as well have been made concerning an actual waking trip as concerning an hallucinated one. The subject insisted that, in giving this report, she referred to her recollection of a very real experience, just as she would if she were recounting a waking event. We have spared no effort to cross-examine subjects on this point and without exception they insist that such is the nature of their mental processes while reporting. Of course, the amount of detail that one spontaneously offers in telling of a past experience varies with the individual and his instructions as well as with what he happened to notice. By asking special questions concerning detail, subjects will supply an additional amount from their recollection of the experience. It is well to point out that in normal life one frequently may not observe a great deal concerning one's physical environment because one's attention may be directed elsewhere.

No other suggestion than that given in Item 3 was used. Yet we see that in this reported activity of the subject's own choosing she and her sister amused themselves by playing an old-fashioned game known as "roadside cribbage", which involves counting. The fact that some of her previous tasks were concerned with counting hallucinatory objects probably explains this. We consider that the counting experiments, which will be described later, are of special significance, for they provide us with a sort of "subjective clock".

Another interesting thing about this report is the presence of what might be termed a "coincidental happening". We refer to the incident of stopping to buy lemonade from the little girl. Such a thing is so typically human and natural that, in our opinion, it lends credence to the subject's report. We have encountered many similar incidents, and shall list a number of them elsewhere.

It need hardly be pointed out that the usual basis we have for an assumption concerning the nature of another individual's experience is some form of communication. This is most commonly effected by means of verbalization, either spoken or written. Spoken words are an auditory phenomenon, and written words a visual one, and both belong to the "public" world. It is obvious therefore that our problem is to evaluate, in terms of her actual experience, our subject's report, and it is upon the answer to this question that the significance of this work depends.

If our subject was deliberately fabricating for any reason whatsoever, or if she was indulging in unconscious fabrication or elaboration, we are in no position to know the nature of her experience during the activity interval.

Another possibility, as will be shown in Chapter 22, is that our suggestion gave rise to a delusion, that is, to the mere belief that she had taken an automobile ride, and that she filled in the descriptive details during her report either consciously or unconsciously. In this connection it is well to remind the reader that in normal waking life a person may remember, and therefore believe rightly, that he has been in a certain place in the past, but he is nonetheless unable to supply any of the details. If our subject were under the delusion that she had taken an automobile ride, that is, if she simply *believed* that she had, and if she was honest and was not indulging in unconscious falsification or elaboration, she would merely state that she could give none of the details although she was certain she took the ride. Actually, this has occurred among our subjects.

In Item 12, the reply "Oh, yes!" was given with obvious emotional feeling.

It is to be hoped that the above brief introduction will induce the reader to entertain in his mind at least the possibility that our subjects' reports are indeed descriptions of real experiences. This may, in the opinion of some persons, be asking a great deal of their credulity, and so it might be appropriate to point out that all of us accept the reality of nocturnal dreams, themselves a naturally occurring form of hallucinatory phenomena which frequently show time distortion. The reason for this general acceptance is undoubtedly the fact that dreams are a common human experience known to each of us. Yet our evidence that other people than ourselves do dream consists solely in verbal reports from the dreamer. True, hallucinatory experience under conditions of time distortion in the trance state has been had by a relatively small number of experimental subjects, but this fact in itself is not an adequate reason for denying to these reports the same status, as far as credibility is concerned, that we grant to reports concerning the common nocturnal dream. We realize, of course, that the experiences alleged by our subjects, when taken in conjunction with their time relations, are astonishing and, on first consideration, somewhat incredible. However, doubts concerning the veracity of such reports must not be based on the amazing nature of their content, but rather on such tendencies towards falsification, elaboration, or delusion production as may be connected with the trance state and the phenomena associated therewith. The possible role played by these and other factors will be discussed at some length in subsequent chapters.

The initial experiments brought up many questions, as indeed did subsequent ones, and this work as a whole is an attempt to answer some of them. The resulting investigations have been less thorough in some instances than in others, and consequently the results vary in significance. We are presenting the less conclusive findings along with the more conclusive ones in the hope that this will stimulate further research in a field that may prove fruitful from the point of view of psychology, psychiatry, and philosophy.

CHAPTER 2

Time

Einstein has made the following statement: "The experiences of an individual appear to us arranged in a series of events; in this series the single events which we remember appear to be ordered according to the criterion of 'earlier' and 'later'. There exists, therefore, for the individual, an I-time, or subjective time. This in itself is not measurable. I can, indeed, associate numbers with the events, in such a way that a greater number is associated with the later event than with an earlier one. This association I can define by means of a clock by comparing the order of events furnished by the clock with the order of the given series of events. We understand by a clock something which provides a series of events which can be counted." (1) (*Also see footnote on page 10.*)

While the hands of a clock move from one position to another, an infinite number of other changes take place in the cosmos. And wherever that phenomenon which we call awareness exists, there is probably a sense of the passage of time, and a sense of sequence. In other words, experience seems to be inseparably interwoven with time sense which, as is true of other "primary" experience, is indefinable. Yet we all know what it is, and we apparently conceive of duration as a magnitude, for we speak of a long or a short time, and readily compare time intervals one with another. Our experience of time differs from that of space in a strange way in that it seems to be *of* us, and inseparable from our very existence.

EXPERIENTIAL TIME

Let us suppose that we gently strike two stones together twice. The two sounds so produced constitute two experiential events which are remembered. Of these sounds we can say:

1. They occurred *simultaneously* with the striking together of the stones.

2. Each was present for only an *instant*.
3. One sound *preceded* the other.
4. Between them there was an *interval* of time.
5. The interval had *duration*.
6. During the interval we were aware of the *passage or flow of time*

All this is known in immediate experience without reference to any sort of a clock, and we refer to the means whereby this is possible as our time sense, or *sense of experiential time*. Our awareness of the "flow" or passage of time is confined to the present and our recollection of this permits us to know duration. Duration is a non-spatial magnitude and, within limits, we can compare the duration of time intervals or events. The shortest perceptible duration is the *instant*, which may be thought of as a point in experiential time. Since duration is a magnitude, points or loci are ordered within it, so that we can know that one instant is earlier or later than another. In other words, the relation sequence is knowable in immediate experience. When two events are experienced at the same instant, we are aware of the relation *simultaneity*. The term *experiential* time, then, in its broader meaning, includes all these concepts. In a narrower usage, it is applied to the feeling of duration.

It is our sense of duration which leads us to think of experiential time intervals as magnitudes. And indeed, short experiential time intervals can be truly compared, within limits, by referring to our sense of duration. Thus we can know in immediate experience that one such interval is longer than another. Furthermore, since our life is regulated by clocks, each of us has a more or less definite idea of the sense of duration we usually experience when the second-hand of a clock moves over one one-second division. This allows us, with fair accuracy, to count at such a rate that the second-hand of a clock moves over one one-second division in the interval between each pair of numbers. These "experiential seconds" might be considered to be true units, though inaccurate ones, of experiential time. The same may be said of "experiential minutes" and small multiples thereof.

Unfortunately, as will be seen below, the word "duration" is used in physics in an entirely different sense. In physics it means the clock reading of a time interval, that is, the advance of clock-hands, measured in spatial units, during an interval.

WORLD TIME

In classical physics a confusing position has been taken concerning the experiential time interval, for here it is stipulated that intervals of experiential time shall be compared by means of the motion of bodies. Thus two such intervals are defined as equal when a body, moving under exactly the same circumstances in both cases, moves as far during one interval as during the other. For practical purposes, the rotation of the earth has been chosen as an instance of motion that continues under "exactly the same circumstances", and so if a point on the earth's surface moves through an arc of the same length during two intervals of experiential time, the intervals are said to be equal. And as our ordinary clocks are calibrated to the rotation of the earth, when a point on a clock hand moves through an arc of the same length during two intervals, the intervals, again, are said to be equal. In experience, motion implies change in position in experiential space and this is measured by means of experiential spatial units. In the case of the minute-hand of a clock, the circle on the dial over which the tip moves is divided into 60 equal arcs called minutes. In the case of the second-hand, the circle is divided into 60 equal arcs called seconds. These arcs, then, are *distances* on the circumference of a circle over which the hand moves. They are experiential spatial units, and the "intervals" between each two minute-marks and each two second-marks are experiential spatial intervals, and not intervals of experiential time. True, if a person notes the instant at which the minute-hand is at the point marked 12, and that at which it is at the point marked 1, he is aware that these two instants are separated by an interval of experiential time. But his sense of duration while the hand moves over these same five minute-divisions may be very different when, an hour later, he repeats the observation, for this sense of duration depends upon many different factors.

In time distortion in hypnosis, there may be a very marked difference in the experiential duration of two time intervals during each of which a clock hand advanced the same distance. The first one may seem to the subject to last one minute, and the second one 30 minutes, depending upon the suggestions given. Yet when compared according to the method of the physicists, the intervals are pronounced equal. Thus our clocks do not truly measure, or compare, quantities of experiential time.

Clock-dial units are, of course, arbitrarily related to the rotation of the earth. While the second-hand of a clock moves over one one-second division, a point on the earth's surface advances by approximately one 86400th part of the circumference of the circle in which it moves. We shall use the term *clock reading* (C.R.) for these clock-dial distances as measured in seconds or minutes, the term *clock* to include the ordinary clock, the watch, or the stop-watch. In the metronome experiments, our metronome was calibrated to a clock. The expression "the rate of the metronome was constant at 60 strokes per minute" means that 60 strokes were sounded while the minute-hand of a clock advanced over one one-minute division on the dial, or that during the experiential time interval between any two successive strokes, the second-hand of a clock advanced over one one-second division.

In summary, the seconds and minutes shown on our clock dial are experiential spatial units, just as are the centimeters or inches on a ruler. They measure difference in the position of a hand resulting from motion during an experiential time interval. It is clear then, that although we refer to them as units of time, it is a time that is quite different from experiential time. Indeed, the word time, as here used, can readily be defined in terms of spatial concepts. We designate this form of time as clock time, physical time, objective time, or *world time* (W.T.).

Footnote to p. 7. Einstein, in the 5th edition of his book "The Meaning of Relativity" (Princeton University Press, 1955) says on page 1, "We understand by a clock something which provides a series of events which can be counted, and which has other properties of which we shall speak later." Then, on page 2, he says, "The conception of physical bodies, in particular of rigid bodies, is a relatively constant complex of such sense perceptions. A clock is also a body, or a system, in the same sense, with the additional property that the series of events which it counts is formed of elements all of which can be regarded as equal".

CHAPTER 3

Definitions

The time of experience. In this work, duration is the most important component of experiential time. However, the sense of the passage or "flow" of time and the temporal relations of sequence and simultaneity are knowable only through our sense of experiential time. This has been discussed in Chapter 2.

WORLD TIME (W.T.)

Synonyms for world time are clock time, physical time, or objective time. This sort of time was discussed in Chapter 2, where it was pointed out that its units are really spatial, and are read from the dial of a clock or watch.

When we speak of the world time of a time interval or event we refer to the clock reading during the event or interval. In such cases, the term world time (W.T.) and clock reading (C.R.) are interchangeable.

When we allot a definite amount of world time to a task, we call this the *allotted time* (A.T.) of the task. Where no allotted time is used, that is, where the subject is instructed to notify us by signal when he has finished a task, we refer to the clock reading between the starting signal and his signal as the world time (W.T.) of the task.

CLOCK READING (C.R.)

The clock reading of a time interval or an event is the distance, measured in seconds or minutes, over which a clock hand has advanced during the interval or event. In other words, it is the number of second-divisions or minute-divisions over which the hand moved during the interval or event.

In some instances we speak of the *"actual duration"* or "world time" of an interval instead of its "clock reading". We prefer "clock reading"

11

to "actual duration" because the term emphasizes the fact that it is an experiential spatial concept.

SEEMING DURATION (S.D.)

This is a person's answer to the question, "How long did it seem?" This question may, of course, refer to an interval, or to an event. An event, unless instantaneous, has a beginning and an end, and thus occupies the interval between these two points in experiential time. In previous publications we have used the term, "Estimated Personal Time (E.P.T.)" for this concept.

We all come to associate, in our minds, a certain quantity of subjective time with a given amount of movement of the clock hands. Thus the term "one second" or "one minute" means not only a certain distance advanced by the clock hands, but likewise a subjective time interval with a certain duration. Indeed, as mentioned above, if we are asked to count out a series of one-second intervals, in the absence of a clock, we can do so with a fair degree of accuracy.

Although we cannot at present accurately measure experiential time, we can gain some idea of the seeming duration of a time interval or of an event by asking a waking person, "How long did it seem?" He might reply that "It seemed a long time" or "It seemed a short time." If we ask him, "How many minutes did it seem to be?" he might reply that the interval *seemed* to be five minutes long. By this he means that his sense of the passage of time during the interval, that is, his sense of its duration, was *approximately that which he generally experiences while the minute-hand of a clock advances over five one-minute divisions,*—i.e. through an arc of 30 degrees. On being informed that the clock hand had advanced by only two minutes, he might reply, "It seemed longer than it was (by the clock)."

Now let us suppose that we ask a waking individual, who has not had access to a clock, how long a certain meeting, which we know to have taken 30 minutes, lasted. He will, before answering, review his experience during the time interval. In fact, he may revise his first answer as he reflects further on the matter.

If he was impatient, uncomfortable, or anxious, his initial estimate may be longer than it would otherwise be. Thus he might say that "It seemed to be a long time, for I was bored and uncomfortable, and impatient to meet someone who was waiting for me." The contrary is likely to be the case if he was interested or absorbed in something, or was enjoying himself.

In the absence of any distinct emotional coloring to his experience, or after he has considered such of this as there was, he may next review what happened during the interval—what he saw or heard or did or thought, etc., and even then he may find conflicting evidence on which to base his judgment. His conclusions, when finally arrived at, may lead to a revision of any that was based on his emotional tone.

In any event, such estimates of the duration of an interval as those just cited constitute the *seeming duration* of the interval, or the *estimated personal time*.

On the other hand, where the person involved finds a "clock-substitute", his answer does not fall in this category. For instance, our friend may later recall that a familiar train was heard to pass just as the meeting started, and another shortly after it ended. This leads him to conclude, rightly, that the meeting probably lasted about a half hour, as he knew when the trains were due to pass by, so that they substituted for a clock.

Again, where a person has the means of actually calculating the advance of a clock during an interval, we no longer consider the result of such a process as an estimate. Thus, a young man who very nearly ran his car over a cliff while taking his fiancée for a drive, reported that the time interval during which they were in danger seemed to be very long. In analyzing certain other aspects of his experience, he told of doing an amount of thinking and reflecting that was appropriate to a long interval. In other words, the seeming duration was long. However, on considering the number of feet which the car had slid with locked wheels and its probable speed when the emergency occurred, he was able to calculate that the clock reading during the emergency was but a few seconds.

Likewise, a frightened parachuter might say that it seemed many minutes before his 'chute opened. In analyzing other aspects of his experience, he might report that, when it finally did open, it did so in a very leisurely fashion, appearing to unfold in "slow motion" as he watched it. Thus, his earlier estimate of the seeming duration was confirmed by visual experience. However, from his knowledge of his altitude, speed of fall, and other factors, he can, by calculation, finally conclude rightly that, during the interval between the pulling of the cord and the opening of the 'chute, the second-hand of a watch advanced over only a few one-second divisions.

In summary, then, we can say that, in the waking state, *seeming duration, or estimated personal time,* is an estimate of the duration of an event or time interval in the absence of a clock, or a clock-substitute, or the necessary data for calculation.

Such an estimate may be given only in vague terms such as "long" or "short". On the other hand, it is often expressed in seconds or minutes. These, of course, are experiential seconds or minutes that he has come to know from past experience.

Now, if we ask a person how long one of his *dreams* seemed to be, his answer will generally be based upon his experience in the dream, and his answer will be in terms of the minutes or hours of his dream-time.

Just as the dreamer has been in a different world, so the hypnotized subject, during hallucinated experience of the type with which we are dealing, has been in a different world. True, in some experiments, we have "injected" sound signals into his hallucinations, but these have fitted into his hallucinated world as part of its fabric.

In asking a subject for a report on a previous hallucinated experience, it is immaterial whether he be still in the trance state, or awake. In either event, in replying to the question, "How long did it seem?" he will generally assume correctly that we are referring to his sense of the passage of time in his hallucinated world. If he doesn't, we can readily explain to him that we are not asking him to estimate how long the experience lasted according to our stop-watch, but how long it seemed to him to last, as he lived it. Once the subject understands this, the actual form in which the question is put is immaterial. We generally use, "How long did it seem?", "How long did it take?", or "How long was it?" He will then go about the answer just as the waking individual went about estimating the duration of his waking experience. And his answer will mean that if the experience had occurred while he was awake, he would have estimated the duration as so many minutes or, had a clock been present in the hallucinated world, its minute-hand would have advanced so far.

TIME DISTORTION

Having defined what we mean by the *seeming duration* of a time interval, which is a concept involving experiential time, and the *clock reading* of a time interval, which involves world time, we shall proceed to a discussion of time distortion. The reader should first be reminded, however, that when a person expresses the seeming duration of a time interval in terms of seconds or minutes, as in saying, "It seemed to last five minutes," he means that he would expect the minute-hand of a clock to advance over five one-minute divisions during the event or interval. This estimate, as pointed out in the previous chapter, is arrived at after reflecting upon various aspects of his experience during the interval or event. In the case of time intervals of very short seeming duration, he need only refer to his idea of the duration of a second, or small multiples thereof.

When the seeming duration of a time interval, expressed in seconds, is markedly different from the clock reading of the same time interval, we say that *time distortion* is present. Mathematically, time distortion is present when the numerical value of the ratio S.D./C.R. (or S.D./W.T.) is considerably larger or smaller than 1. Incidentally, in these experiments we are interested in producing ratios with a numerical value greater than 1.

It is obvious that, under ordinary waking conditions, one's estimate of an interval of experiential time, that is, its seeming duration, is rarely in exact agreement with the clock reading of the interval. Generally, it is either somewhat greater or somewhat less. We reserve the term *time distortion* for those cases where the discrepancy is a large one and consequently where the sense of duration is far out of its usual proportion to the clock reading. The relation thus is a distorted one, and we can refer to the experiential time of the person involved as *distorted time*. An extreme example is the case where a hypnotized subject experiences an hour's hallucinatory activity in, say, a three-second reading on our stopwatch.

It is at once evident that the concept *time distortion* involves two constituent concepts, the *seeming duration* and *clock reading* of a given experiential time interval, and cannot be known until we have determined both of these constituents. A person who has had a narrow escape and has experienced a long seeming duration during the time interval occupied by the event, can conclude that time distortion was present only after he has learned that the clock reading of the interval was very much shorter than the seeming duration. Likewise, in our experiments with hypnotized subjects, we can conclude that time distortion was present only after we have compared the clock reading of an hallucinatory experience with the subject's report of its seeming duration.

In the waking individual, time distortion is a fairly common experience. As mentioned above, intervals with the same clock reading may have a very short seeming duration during pleasure and amusement, or interest, and a very long one during boredom, anticipation, discomfort, or anxiety. This finds expression in such folk sayings as "Time flies on love's wings," or "The watched pot never boils."

In previous papers, where the seeming duration of an interval is much longer than the clock reading, as in the case of the "watched pot", we have said that time was "slowed", for "The minutes seemed to drag by," so to speak. Some persons, on the other hand, thinking of time as a flowing stream, take the view that this is really a "speeding up" of time, for a larger segment of the stream has passed by during the given clock reading of the interval than would ordinarily be the case. Confusion can be avoided by dropping the terms "slowing" or "speeding up" of time, and merely stating whether the ratio of the seeming duration to the clock reading (S.D./C.R.) or to the world time (S.D./W.T.) of the interval is increased or decreased in time distortion. As mentioned above, all the work reported in this monograph deals with a deliberate *increase* in this ratio.

Time distortion is very common in dreams, where many hours of dream-life may be experienced in but a few minutes by the clock. Another type of time distortion, and a most interesting one, may be encountered in times of danger or narrow escape, where intervals of very brief clock reading seem to be long. In such cases, the long seeming duration, or subjective time interval, may be filled with thoughts and images proceeding at an apparently normal rate, and movement in the "physical world", often very rapid in terms of clock time, may appear to the victim to occur in "slow motion". It is by no means rare for the individual involved to report that, in the emergency, his performance was improved because he seemed to have more time for decisions. Again, persons who have nearly drowned have reported reliving large segments of their lives in what proved to be but a few minutes. Such experience proceeds at a normal rate as far as the victim is concerned.

One psychiatrist,[1] who was in an automobile that skidded off the road and that turned completely over twice before landing at the bottom of a decline, commented about his subjective feeling that time was now either standing still or going in slow motion; it seemed to him as though it took approximately half an hour from the time the car started to turn over till it hit the decline on the side, as though it took another half an hour before the car turned over to its roof, as though there was still another half an hour before it turned over to the other side, etc.—and since it turned over two full times in all, as though in the short space of less than a few seconds, over two hours had passed.

The sense of duration may be altered also by organic brain lesions, certain drugs, the psychoses and psychoneuroses, delirium, and toxic states. In general, time seems to pass more rapidly for the aging than for the young.

Welch (20) has made a study of time distortion in hypnotically-induced dreams, and Erickson (9) has reported the phenomenon in a hypnotized

---

[1] Dr. Harold Rosen, in a personal communication.

subject who was reliving past events. Inglis (10) had a subject who claimed to be able to bring about an apparent slowing of observed physical phenomena at will, and to have employed this ability to advantage while boxing, when it aided him in placing blows.

Finally, time sense can be deliberately altered by hypnotic suggestion and a predetermined degree of distortion thus effected.

Depending upon the circumstances, certain other changes in experience may accompany time distortion. The following outline presents some of the more important of these:

Boredom

The ratio between the seeming duration and the clock reading of an interval is increased.

Sensory experience:

No change in apparent speed of progression.

Non-sensory experience:

No change in apparent speed of progression.

The dream

The ratio between the seeming duration and the clock reading of an interval is increased.

Sensory experience from the physical world:

Physical stimuli are usually not experienced as such.

Dream experience:

Much activity may take place in an interval of very brief clock reading. This activity appears, to the subject, to proceed at a normal or customary rate.

Hypnosis

With the proper technique, the ratio between the seeming duration and the clock reading of an interval may be greatly increased, and in a controlled way.

Sensory experience from the physical world:

In the few cases where two sounds have been injected into hallucinatory experiences, the ratio between the seeming duration of the interval and its clock reading has been increased.

Where a single continuous sound has been so injected, its S.D./C.R. ratio has likewise been increased.

Hallucinatory and non-sensory experience:

Much activity may take place in an interval of very brief clock reading. This activity appears, to the subject, to proceed at a normal or customary rate.

The narrow escape

The ratio between the seeming duration and the clock reading of an interval may be greatly increased.

Sensory experience:

    All sensory experience may seem to be slowed down, action appearing to occur in "slow motion". Actually, high speeds in the physical world are often involved.

Non-sensory experience:

    Thought, imagery, etc., are often much increased in amount per unit of world time. As far as the person involved is concerned, the activity seems to proceed at a normal rate.

PERSONAL TIME (P.T.)

Subjective, experiential, or psychological time.

SUGGESTED PERSONAL TIME (S.P.T.)

This is a time interval, or a duration, that is suggested to the subject under hypnosis and which, in a good subject, becomes the time of his experience. It is generally used in connection with a continuous activity, by telling the subject that he will engage in it for a certain length of time. Of course, subjects come to realize, during a series of experiments, that the seeming duration of their hallucinated activities has been different from the reading shown by the experimenter's watch.

TASK OR ACTIVITY

When we make an affirmation to a hypnotized subject concerning himself we are giving him a suggestion, and his response will be to have certain experiences. Similar effects may be produced by giving him a command. His response will, of course, depend upon many factors, among them his own past experience and his understanding of what is said to him.

When we suggest to the subject that he be some place, or do something, we say that we are assigning to him an activity. His response, in either case, involves a change in his field of awareness. This response may involve the hallucinatory production of those forms of experience that make up, in the waking state, the so-called "physical world". Likewise, other forms of sensation may be produced, as well as feeling, emotion, thought, etc.

Obviously, the variety of assignable experiences is almost limitless. If we simply suggest that he *be* somewhere, what he *does* in his hallucinated world is entirely up to him. If we specify that he *do* something, such as take a walk, change a tire on his car, play some game, buy a pair of shoes, listen to a record, watch a set of tennis, think over some problem, etc., he still has a wide field to choose from, including the time and the place of the activity. The suggestion that a subject "take a walk" is more general, or less specific, than that he "take a walk in downtown Washington", while the suggestion that he relive a certain experience is a highly specific one. By using a suggested personal time, we can, within limits, control the seeming duration of a task.

There is a difference between watching baseball, ironing clothes, or counting gum-drops, on the one hand, and watching three innings of a baseball game, ironing six shirts, or counting 100 gum-drops, on the other. The former activities could theoretically continue more or less indefinitely, whereas the latter are, by definition, circumscribed. We call them continuous and completed activities, respectively.

1. Continuous activity: A continuous activity is one which progresses to no stipulated limit as far as definition of the activity itself is concerned. In these experiments, continuous activities are generally limited, in seeming duration, by assigning to them a suggested personal time (S.P.T.). Examples are: walking for ten minutes, picking flowers for half an hour, listening to music for five minutes, etc.

2. Completed activity: A completed activity is one which progresses to the fulfillment of certain stipulated or implied conditions (none of them concerning the duration), at which point it reaches completion. Thus it is self-limited. Examples are: to change a tire, to count a given number of objects, to walk a certain distance, etc.

It will be noted that we have defined the completed activity as being limited by considerations other than duration. This is done in order to permit a special treatment of the time factor.

STARTING SIGNAL

The signal for the hallucinated activity to begin.

TERMINATION SIGNAL

The signal, given by the experimenter, for the hallucinated activity to cease, or, in the case of tasks with no allotted time, the signal, given by the subject, that such activity has ceased.

ALLOTTED TIME (A.T.)

When the experimenter designates, by signal, the time at which the subject is to begin a task and that at which he is to end it, we say that the interval between the signals is the *allotted time*, and refer to the first signal as the *starting signal* and the second as the *termination signal*. The allotted time is the clock reading of the world time and is *never* told to the subject during an experiment. It is evident at once that this is a different technique from one where the experimenter gives the starting signal, but where the subject himself indicates the completion of the task by signalling such completion to the experimenter. The use of an allotted time, of course, permits the experimenter accurately to control the ratio between the seeming duration and the world time in tasks where a suggested personal time is used and accepted. It also permits him to control the ratio between the amount of activity, as implied by the particular task assigned, and the world time.

It was while experimenting with the allotted time that a most interesting and inexplicable finding came to light. A description of these experiments follows. The letter E refers to the experimenter; S to the subject.

1. Task A: First the following task was assigned. Since it proceeds to a stipulated limit (the picking of four rows of cotton), it is a completed task. There is no suggested personal time, for nothing was said to the subject concerning how long she was to work. She was told to signal when she was finished, and hence there was no allotted time.

> E. You are in a cotton field, and are going to pick some cotton. Tell me, please, what you see.
>
> S. (The subject described a cotton field.)
>
> E. Stay there, and listen to me carefully. When I give you the starting signal by saying "Now", you will pick four rows of cotton, counting the bolls as you pick them, one at a time. You will not hurry. When you've finished, you'll let me know by raising your right hand. Here comes the starting signal, "Now".

The subject raised her right hand 217 seconds after the starting signal had been given, and reported that she had picked 719 cotton bolls. She picked with her right hand part of the time, and with her left hand part of the time, shifting the bag accordingly. She picked only ripe bolls, leaving the green ones alone. Sometimes she stopped and brushed the leaves aside to make sure that she hadn't missed any. She didn't hurry, but she worked steadily. It was late afternoon, and the woods along the west edge of the field cast a shadow. She stated that she seemed to have been working about an hour and twenty minutes. When asked to demonstrate, by counting aloud, the rate at which she picked the cotton, she counted to 56 in one minute.

2. Task B: The following task was then assigned. Note that whereas Task A was a completed activity, without an allotted time or a suggested personal time, Task B is a continuous activity since it is, in itself, unlimited. The allotted time was three seconds, and the suggested personal time one hour and twenty minutes.

E. You are now in a cotton field and are going to pick some cotton. Tell me what you see.

S. (The subject described a cotton field.)

E. Stay there and listen to me carefully. When I give you the starting signal by saying "Now", you are going to pick cotton for an hour and twenty minutes. You will not hurry, and you will count each boll as you pick it. Here comes the starting signal, "Now".

(Three seconds later.)

E. Now make your mind a blank. Your mind is now a blank. Tell me what happened, please.

S. (The subject reported that she had picked and counted 862 cotton bolls, one at a time. Again, she had not hurried, but worked steadily. From time to time, she brushed the leaves aside to make sure that she hadn't missed any. It was very "real" and was comparable to her performance in the previous task. Asked how long it seemed, she replied, "An hour and twenty minutes." Asked to demonstrate, by counting aloud, the rate at which she picked the cotton, she counted to 68 in one minute.)

It was this report on Task B, indicating as it did that the subject had approximately the same "amount" of experience in three seconds as she had previously had in 217 seconds, that led us to investigate further the relations between the amount of activity and the allotted time. Furthermore, it revealed the allotted time as one of the most important concepts involved.

In the terminology presented above, the tasks may be described as follows:

Task	A.T.	Completed	Contin-uous	S.P.T.	W.T.	S.D.	D.R.	Count
A	0	+	0	0	217 sec.	80 min.	56/min.	719
B	3 sec.	0	+	+	3 sec.	80 min.	68/min.	862

DEMONSTRATED RATE (D.R.)

In the counting experiments, the subject was frequently asked to demonstrate, by counting out loud, the rate at which he had counted hallucinated objects. This was done both during trance and post-hypnotically. In the former instances, the subject had finished the task and was presumably not in a phase of response to suggestion.

(D.R.)(S.D.)

This product, demonstrated rate multiplied by seeming duration, is a product used in the counting tasks. It indicates the count that would be reached if the subject counted at the demonstrated rate for a period equal to the estimated personal time.

(D.R.)(W.T.)

This product, demonstrated rate multiplied by world time, gives us the count that would be reached if the subject counted at the demonstrated rate for a period equal to the world time.

EXPERIENTIAL SPACE

The space of experience. We say, for instance, that the contents of our visual field are ordered and extended in experiential space. Spatial relations likewise are immediately knowable in auditory and tactile and some other forms of experience and we can correlate some of these sense-specific spaces into a more general one. Thus we can locate a certain sound in relation to a certain portion of our visual field.

CONCURRENT REPORTING

The reporting, by the subject, of his hallucinated activity while it is actually proceeding. It has been used by us very rarely, the most frequent occasion being as a prelude to some of the counting experiments.

CHAPTER 4

Subjects

Pertinent data concerning the subjects used in these experiments is presented below:

TABLE 1

SUBJECT	AGE	SEX	MARITAL STATUS	EDUCATION	OCCUPATION
A	40	F	M	?	Housewife
B	36	F	S	High school	Secretary
C	25	M	M	College	Student
D	23	F	M	College	Student
E	23	F	S	College	Student
F	32	F	M	College	Teacher
G	18	F	M	High school	Housewife
H	28	M	M	College	Student
I	22	M	S	College	Student
J	19	M	S	High school	Student
K	23	F	S	High school	Typist
L	25	M	M	High school	Building maintenance
M	36	F	M	High school	Secretary
N	20	F	S	College	Student

Subjects C, E, H, I and M were psychology students.

CHAPTER 5

Methods

In this chapter, certain methods of more or less general application will be described. Those that are limited to a particular group of experiments will be considered in the appropriate sections.

In all the experiments, a task was assigned to the hypnotized subject, and the relation between the *seeming duration* and the *clock reading* of the experience was studied, along with certain aspects of the experience itself. The seeming duration, and a description of the experience, were determined by asking the subject for a report. The clock reading was taken from a stop-watch or in some instances it was calculated from a metronome.

Subjects either lay supine on a bed, or sat in a chair, with their eyes closed. It is important to point out that they remained motionless throughout, regardless of what they were doing in their hallucinated world. During the early training sessions, we generally told the subject to *imagine* that he was living the suggested experience. This conveyed to him the idea that we did not expect any motor performance in the "physical" world.

Very occasionally, during early training, some motion may be observed during hallucinatory activity. This can be prevented by suggesting to the subject that, during task performance, regardless of what he does in the hallucinated world, his "physical" body, as opposed to the body which engages in the hallucinatory activity, will remain motionless. Although such a statement may be theoretically ambiguous, the subject invariably knows what the experimenter means by it, and responds accordingly.

Induction of a simple trance state was effected by suggestions of sleep. In general, a moderately deep trance state was quite satisfactory, but there were, of course, individual variations in this regard. Except in special instances, subjects who showed a tendency to develop an amnesia were given the suggestion that they would remember their experiences.

If it was felt advisable to clear the subject's mind of residual scenes before starting an experiment, he was told, "Now, any scenes that you've been seeing are disappearing from view. They have now disappeared, and your mind is now a blank."

Sessions were generally held four or five days a week, in quiet surroundings, and usually lasted an hour.

Each individual experiment consists of the following components:

INTRODUCTION

We generally use the expression, "Now, give me your attention, please. When I give you the starting signal, by saying 'Now', you're going to (you will) . . . ."

ACTIVITY INSTRUCTIONS

Here instructions are given to the subject concerning the experience that he is to have. They may be general or specific, according to the wishes of the experimenter. A list of typical activity instructions follows:

Continuous Activities without Suggested Personal Time:
"... go walking."
"... be in the country, picking blackberries."
"... be listening to a record."
"... take the pennies out of the box, and place them on the table and count them, one by one, as you do so."
"... be in a theater, watching a show."
"... go in swimming."
"... go on a picnic."
"... be at a party."
"... be at work."
"... go shopping."
"... be at an amusement park."
"... be at a dance."

Completed Activities without Suggested Personal Time:
"... prepare a meal."
"... buy a pair of shoes."
"... watch a movie 'short'. "
"... take a walk."
"... draw a picture."
"... watch a set of tennis."

"... do something which you will enjoy."
"... make your bed."
"... change a tire on your car."
"... write a letter."
"... discuss some matter with a friend."
"... have your hair cut."
"... be 8 years old, and will leave your house and walk to school."

If a suggested personal time is used, it is assigned along with the activity instructions. This is generally done in one of the following ways:

"You're going to (you will) spend (at least) 10 minutes (of your special time) watching a baseball game."
"You're going to (you will) be watching a baseball game. You will do this for (at least) 10 minutes (of your special time)."

The term "at least", which is optional, gives a certain leeway to the subject.

Subjects come to think of the time of their hallucinatory experiences as being different from that of the waking world, just as is the time experienced in dreams. This, indeed, is true, and it is often useful to encourage this point of view during training, as is pointed out in Chapter 6. When a subject is helped by this concept, we are likely to use the phrase, "of your special time", after a designated time interval.

Examples of activity instructions with an assigned suggested personal time follow:

Continuous Activities with Suggested Personal Time:
"... go walking for 10 minutes."
"... be in the country picking blackberries. You will do this for (at least) 10 minutes."
"... listen to a record for 5 minutes."
"... pick flowers in a garden for 15 minutes."
"... spend (at least) 10 minutes of your special time taking the pennies out of the box and placing them on the table. You will count them, one by one, as you do so."
"... spend 10 minutes in a theater, watching a show."
"... be at a picnic for half an hour."
"... spend (at least) 20 minutes of your special time at a party."

Completed Activities with Suggested Personal Time:

These are seldom used, for the assigning of a completed activity implies an appropriate experiential time.

"... prepare a meal. It will take an hour."

"... buy a pair of shoes. It will take 20 minutes."

"... watch a movie 'short'. It will take 10 minutes."

Time distortion is aided by assuring the subject that he will have all the time he needs and that he will not have to hurry. Subjects state that such assurance enables them to relax and, unless one is dealing with a very proficient subject, it is advisable to make use of this technique frequently. We use such suggestions as the following:

"You will not have to hurry, for you will have all the time you need."

"Don't hurry; *take your time.*"

"Remember, you have an unlimited amount of special time available and will take as much of this as you need to finish the task without hurrying."

"You will do this slowly, for you will have all the time you need."

"Loiter over this task; *do it slowly.*"

"Relax and take things easy. There's no need to hurry."

"You will complete the task, without hurrying, for you will have plenty of time."

The above type of suggestion is very effective, and frequently enables a subject to finish a completed activity in a leisurely manner, within the allotted time, whereas previously he had been unable to do so.

It is important to point out that we do not tell the subject the allotted time, and that we never give any suggestion to him that will convey any idea related to hurrying or the rapid progression of events. In fact, as stressed above, we give him every assurance that he will have plenty of time and will not have to hurry. This is emphasized because some experimenters, not fully understanding the concept of time distortion, have given suggestions to the effect that experiences will "flash" or "rush" through the subject's mind. This, of course, is just the opposite result to that which we aim for. True, if the experimenter could himself observe the events in his subject's mind as they unfold under the type of time distortion described in this report—that is, where the S.D./C.R. ratio is much larger than 1—the activity would be found to proceed at a very rapid rate in terms of world time. But we are not interested in this hypothetical finding in giving our suggestion. Rather, we are interested in inducing in the subject experience that progresses at a *normal or natural rate* as far as he is concerned and that is accompanied by a sense of duration appropriate to this rate. That we are successful is evidenced by the subjects' reports.

The writing of notes on a report, or the planning for a subsequent task may, of course, take several minutes. In such cases, we generally say to the subject, "Now let your mind wander whither it will, to pleasant scenes." This permits him to engage in desultory hallucinatory activity of his own choosing, and allows him to relax. When we are ready to assign the next task, we say, "Now give me your attention, please. Any scenes you've been seeing are now disappearing from view. Your mind is now a blank."

During long sessions, it is our custom to allow the subject to refresh himself by assigning to him the following task: "You will spend as much time as you wish doing something that you will enjoy." In the case of accomplished subjects, an allotted time of 20 or 30 seconds is used for this "recess". With other subjects, it is longer.

STARTING SIGNAL

This is simply the word, "Now".

ACTIVITY INTERVAL

This is the period between the starting and the termination signals, during which the subject performs the assigned task. Its clock reading is the same as the allotted time (A.T.) when such is used. When no allotted time is used, it is the same as the world time (W.T.) of the activity.

TERMINATION SIGNAL

a. In the presence of an allotted time (A.T.), the termination of the activity is, of course, brought about by the experimenter. It is explained to the subject that when the experimenter wishes him to terminate the hallucinatory activity, he will say, "Now, make your mind a blank," or "Now, blank." He is told that this constitutes the "termination signal" for all tasks in which the experimenter gives such a signal, and that, when it is given, all hallucinatory activity will stop immediately.

Having explained to the subject that he will receive both a starting and a termination signal, the following suggestions are given after the activity instructions:

(1) With a continuous activity with a suggested personal time
"I shall give the termination signal when the time is up."
(2) With a completed activity
"you will have plenty of time, between signals, to complete the
task without hurrying."

In this work, we use an allotted time with almost all the tasks. Consequently, our subjects come to expect the termination signal as a matter of course. Thus, in trained subjects, it is unnecessary to say anything, routinely, about the termination signal when an allotted time is used.

b. In the absence of an allotted time (A.T.), and when the suggested activity is a completed one, the subject is instructed to notify the experimenter when he has finished the task. He is told, "When you've finished, you will let me know by saying, 'Now'." This is also done with continuous activities without an allotted time, which are always given a suggested personal time (S.P.T.) in these experiments.

REPORT

During the early experiments, we requested a report from the subject immediately after the completion of a given task, and while he was still in the trance state. He was then waked, and a waking report was obtained. As these were always in agreement, it became our custom to omit the trance report. Thus, a number of tasks could be assigned and reported upon in a single trance session.

The following expressions are used in obtaining general reports:

"Tell me what happened, please."
"Now, tell me about it."
"Tell me what you did."
"What happened?"
"What did you do?"

Other questions are then asked, such as:

"How long did it seem?"
"Did you finish?"
"Was it real?"
"Did you hurry?"
"Were there any omissions or gaps?"
"Did you enjoy it?"

The following suggestion is generally used in waking the subject: "I'm going to wake you now by counting to 5. When I reach 5 you'll be wide awake and refreshed, and will remember everything you've done. Here comes the waking count—One, you're waking, waking, waking. Two, you're waking, etc." It is important to point out that, except for the instructions that the subject will remember his experiences, nothing is ever said to the subject that would fall in the category of a post-hypnotic suggestion. In other words, post-hypnotic suggestions, except for the instance just noted, are scrupulously avoided.

In the tabulation of results, code designations are built up from the following symbols:

A.T.0: no allotted time was used.
A.T.+: an allotted time was used.
A: a continuous activity.
B: a completed activity.
1: no mention is made of the duration of the activity.
2: the subject is told, "You'll have plenty of time," or is given a similar suggestion.
3: a definite suggested personal time (S.P.T.) is assigned.

Thus A.T.0, A1 means that no allotted time was used, that the activity was continuous, and that no stipulation was made concerning its duration.

CLASSIFICATION OF ACTIVITY INSTRUCTIONS

I. Without allotted time
  Continuous activity
    Without suggested personal time (Code A.T.0, A1)
      "You're going to go walking." (This type of activity was not used in these experiments, as it would tend to continue indefinitely.)
    With suggested personal time (Code A.T.0, A3)
      "You're going to walk for 10 minutes."
  Completed activity
    Without suggested personal time (Code A.T.0, B1)
      "You're going to draw a picture."
    With suggested personal time (Code A.T.0, B3)
      "You're going to spend 10 minutes drawing a picture."

II. With allotted time
    Continuous activity
        Without suggested personal time (Code A.T.+, A1)
        "You're going to go walking."
        With suggested personal time (Code A.T.+, A3)
        "You're going to spend 10 minutes walking."
    Completed activity
        Without suggested personal time (Code A.T.+, B1)
        "You're going to draw a picture."
        With suggested personal time (Code A.T.+, B3)
        "You're going to spend 10 minutes drawing a picture."

CHAPTER 6

Training

In this section, those techniques will be considered whereby a subject, already trained in the production of the more common phenomena characteristic of the trance state, is taught to experience time distortion and to perform the various sorts of tasks discussed in this treatise.

Although a small percentage of "good" subjects will produce many of the phenomena under discussion on the first attempt to elicit them, it is most important for investigators to realize that the training of subjects for time distortion in hypnosis usually requires considerable time, effort, and skill. Methods that succeed with one subject may fail with another, and a keen appreciation of, and sensitivity to, the delicate interpersonal relationship involved in hypnosis is of paramount importance, along with resourcefulness, and the willingness to try original and varying approaches. By and large, training in time distortion requires from three to 20 hours (best spent in daily sessions), not including the time required for the training in hypnosis per se. Furthermore, once learned, the ability decreases with lack of use and retraining may then be necessary to restore the former level of proficiency. With sufficient effort, and the proper technique, the phenomenon can probably be produced, to varying degrees, in the majority of subjects. A casual approach to the work is almost certain to lead to disappointment.

In general, it may be said that time distortion, and related phenomena, depends upon a high degree of withdrawal, by the subject, into his hallucinated world, with an accompanying lack of awareness of his surroundings as such. This state of detachment, in which the subject becomes completely engrossed in his hallucinatory experience, constitutes the first goal in training. When achieved, subjects will report that, during their task performance, they were quite unaware of their surroundings. Indeed, some subjects have reported that, at the termination signal, they experienced a slight "jolt" or "shock". One subject gave evidence of her engrossment in a different world by referring to the termination of the task by saying, "When you *called me out*, I was combing my hair." When

32

she said this, she was still in the trance state, reporting on the performance of a just-completed task. Sudden noises likewise will "jolt" a subject who is hallucinating during time distortion, and sometimes they will destroy the production.

A most helpful suggestion to encourage withdrawal from the physical world is, "During these experiences you will be completely unaware of your surroundings in the waking world."

Prior to the starting signal, while the experimenter is assigning the task, subjects generally think about what they will do. Then, with the starting signal, well-trained subjects find themselves in the hallucinated world, living the assigned experience. This may or may not proceed along the lines they had planned, but it generally satisfies the conditions stipulated in the instructions, and is subject to volitional direction by the subject. Thus, not only does he do what was suggested to him but, within this limitation, he will carry out decisions as he is faced with them, just as he does when awake. One subject, for instance, whose wrist became uncomfortable while hallucinating the writing of a large amount of material, interrupted the writing long enough to go into the bathroom and put some alcohol on the lame wrist (this was, of course, hallucinatory activity only, and involved no actual movement).

The well-trained subject does not consciously construct the details of his hallucinated world, but rather finds himself among them. In other words, whatever be the mechanism of phantasy production, it is spontaneous and effortless. This is in sharp contrast to the case of the waking subject who is asked, say, to imagine that he is looking at his house. Here he is likely deliberately to construct the image from his knowledge of it, and this is accompanied by more or less effort, depending upon how good a visualizer he is. And even then his productions generally lack what Dunne refers to as "reality tone", which is so characteristic of hallucinatory experience. One of our subjects exemplified this in describing how he went about putting himself into a self-induced trance state. He said, "I first imagine myself in a certain situation as, for instance, lying on a rubber raft off a beach. I look about me and visualize the raft, the water, and so forth, and imagine that I feel the warm sun on my back and hear the waves. After a while, *everything comes into focus*, and I'm 'actually there'."

We have always used the word "Now" as a starting and termination signal, and have avoided concurrent reporting almost entirely. Concurrent reporting is the reporting on an experience, by the subject, as he is actually living it, and is, of course, common practice in experimental hypnosis. We avoid it because we believe that it tends to prevent the subject from becoming detached from his surroundings in the physical world, and hence from learning time distortion. Obviously, experience proceeding in distorted time cannot be reported concurrently, for it proceeds too rapidly relative to world time.

It would seem that reality tone is in some way dependent upon a free flow of material from the unconscious. Since most persons dream, it may be well to cite dreams, pointing out to the subject that they are a form of hallucinatory experience, that they show reality tone and time distortion, and that the dreamer is quite unaware of his surroundings. This will give him an idea of the sort of thing that we are after. And in order to encourage a free and spontaneous flow of material from the unconscious, it is probably advisable to instruct the subject to permit free association to guide his imagery during his early training. Some such suggestion as the following may be used:

"When I give you the starting signal by saying, 'Now', you will let some sort of visual image, or scene, come to you. It makes no difference what it is. As you watch, other images will come, of their own accord, one after another. These images will become more and more clear and more and more real, so that eventually you will find yourself 'actually there' in another world. You will be a part of that world, which will be just as real as the waking world, and you will truly *live* such experiences as you have there. After a while I shall say to you, 'Now, make your mind a blank', whereupon all hallucinatory activity will cease. I shall then ask you to tell me what you saw or did, but you need tell me only what you wish of your experience."

The subject is thus introduced to the use of a starting signal and a termination signal.

The subject should be allowed several minutes (allotted time) for such an exercise.

The next step is to assign definite tasks. These tasks should be familiar ones, and the instructions should be as general as possible. This permits the subject a wide range of action, with a minimum of limitations. We may simply instruct him to do anything he wishes. At first we may tell him that he is to *imagine* himself in such a place, or doing such and such a thing. Soon we discontinue the use of the phrase "to imagine" and tell him that he *will be* in such a place, or *will do* so and so, adding that "it will be very real, so that you will actually live the experience."

As training progresses, a series of tasks are run with completed activities. In these, it is important to assure the subject, after the activity suggestion, that he will "have plenty of time between signals to complete the task". In order to be certain that the allotted time is long enough for him so to complete the task, it may be assigned first with no allotted time, allowing the subject to signal when he has finished. Having noted the world time, the task is then repeated, using the world time as the allotted time. By employing this technique with a number of tasks, the subject is introduced to the use of completed activities that he can finish within an allotted time.

Examples of such tasks follow:

"When I give you the starting signal by saying 'Now', you will . . .
". . . take a walk."
". . . buy a pair of shoes."
". . . watch a movie 'short'."
". . . order a meal in a restaurant."
". . . draw a picture."
". . . polish your shoes."
". . . change a tire on a car."
". . . hear a record."

Here again, a report of each task, with its seeming duration, should be obtained.

Early in training, the seeming duration may be way out of proportion to the amount of activity reported. As the work progresses, this disproportion tends to disappear, and the amount of activity becomes more appropriate to the experiential time.

Next, continuous activities with a suggested personal time and an allotted time are introduced. The "finishing" of such activities consists, of course, in the activity having continued for the suggested personal time. Here again, it may be well to run the activity first as a task without an allotted time, allowing the subject to signal when he has finished. It can then be repeated, using the world time interval as the allotted time. With this, the subject should be assured that "when the time (suggested personal time) is up, the termination signal will be given." These activities are introduced by telling the subject that he will be at a certain place, or doing a certain thing. The reliving of pleasant past experiences is a type of task that is useful at this stage of training. However, any familiar type of activity is quite satisfactory, such as the following:

"When I give you the starting signal by saying 'Now', you will . . .
". . . be at a beach."
". . . be in the country."

"... be in school."
"... be at work."
"... be on a vacation."
"... be taking a walk."
"... be at a movie."
"... be taking a drive in a car."
etc.

The subject should be asked for a report after each task, and the seeming duration of the experience should be asked for. Time distortion will soon become evident to the experimenter and, at some point in the training, it is advisable to point out to the subject the difference between the seeming duration and the clock reading during his experiences. This will help him to realize that time distortion is a fact, and that he himself can experience it quite naturally. In this way, the subject will become accustomed to finishing "completed" activities and "continuous" ones (with a suggested personal time) within an allotted time.

The next step is to run a series of tasks, either completed or continuous (with suggested personal time), using at first an allotted time long enough to permit the subject to finish the task and then, in repeating it, gradually to decrease the allotted time in steps of from 10 to 30 seconds. The subject, "caught short" at first, will soon learn to adjust to the shorter allotted time, and will fit his hallucinatory experience into the interval allowed him, without hurrying, or compromising in any way. Thus he learns to work with short allotted times. How far the process can be carried is not known at present.

A few words are in order concerning suggested personal time. This is used, as a rule, only with continuous activities, and may be introduced by such an expression as, "You will spend 10 minutes (of your special time) doing so and so." Or, the experimenter may say, after the activity instructions, "You will do this for 10 minutes."

Some subjects readily accept this early in their training; others have difficulty doing so. The difficulty seems to arise from at least two factors—a residual awareness of surroundings and consequently of world time, and a deep conviction that it "just is impossible". Practice, and use of a deeper trance, will help overcome the first difficulty. With the second, it may help to point out to the subject that he has on many occasions during his training himself experienced the variability of subjective time in relation to world time. The results of some of his earlier tests will convince him of this when shown to him.

Repeated assurance, to the subject, that he will have plenty of time for his task is of great importance during training, and should be used frequently. Such suggestions should be given with conviction, and it is often wise to repeat them many times. Examples are:

"You will have plenty of time."
"You will not have to hurry."
"You will have all the time you need."
"Relax and take your time."
"You can loiter over it if you wish."
"Remember, you have an unlimited supply of special trance time at your disposal, so take as much of it as you need."
"You are to do this slowly, without hurrying."

We have found the following technique useful, at times, in teaching the subject to work with short allotted times. It consists merely in suggesting a series of 10 tasks, each with an allotted time of 10 seconds, with reporting deferred until the series has been completed.

0 sec.: "When I give you the starting signal by saying 'Now', you will get a haircut. . .
10 sec.: "Now."
20 sec.: "Now, blank. At the next signal you will wash your car. . .
30 sec.: "Now."
40 sec.: "Now, blank. At the next signal you will buy a pair of shoes. . .
50 sec.: "Now."
etc.

Another helpful technique is to repeat a given task over and over, keeping the allotted time constant. Although the subject may not be able to finish it at first, he often will learn to do so, without hurrying in the slightest, after repeated attempts. This will facilitate high degrees of time distortion in subsequent tasks.

To encourage progress, the activity instruction should be followed by such suggestions as the following, given repeatedly, and with conviction:

"You will finish this, without hurrying."
"Remember, you're going to finish this task, and you won't hurry."
"You will take as much time as you need to finish the task without hurrying."
"You will finish the task."

A most interesting technique, learned from Erickson and applicable to a very wide range of suggestions is, after an affirmatory suggestion, to ask the subject the question, "Won't you?" thus:

"You will finish, won't you?"

The subject, in answering "Yes," increases the likelihood of his carrying out the suggestion.

This technique may be used with commands in the following way:

"Take as much time as you need in order to finish the task. You'll do this, won't you?"

Even further affirmatory reinforcement may be obtained by adding, "Are you sure?" after the subject has answered "Yes" to the above question.

As is pointed out elsewhere, the hallucinatory productions with which we deal in these experiments are, in certain important respects, different from most dreams. On the other hand, the nocturnal dream is the commonest form of experience that resembles them, and in which time distortion is present. Therefore, in some subjects, production of a few hypnotically-induced dreams may serve as a useful introduction to hallucinatory experience of the sort we seek to develop. If dreams are produced, we explain to the subject that we shall ask for no more of them, but shall strive for productions that are identical with waking experience, that are continuous, "real" experiences, which he will actually *live*. Thus they will "make sense", will be rich in detail, and will contain no omissions or gaps. We must frequently suggest that the experiences will be "very, very real, so that you will actually live them". This is extremely important.

At some point during training, it is desirable to discuss time with the subject. How this is done will vary with different experimenters. We generally employ some such approach as the following:

"There are two kinds of time: one, the time the clock tells us, the other, our own sense of the passage of time. The first of these is known as physical, or solar, or world time. It is the time used by the physicists and the astronomers in their measurements, and by all of us in our work-a-day life. The second is called personal, or subjective time. Einstein refers to this as 'I-time'.

"It is this subjective time that we are most interested in here. One of the most important things about it is that it is very variable. Thus, if several persons are asked to judge the length of a five minute interval as measured by a clock, they may have very different ideas as to the duration of the interval, depending upon the circumstances in which each person finds himself. To those who were enjoying themselves, or who were absorbed in some interesting activity, the interval might well seem shorter. On the other hand, to those in pain or discomfort, or anxiety, the five minutes would seem much longer. We call this time distortion, and the most familiar example of it is found in the dream. You yourself have probably often noticed that you can experience many hours of dream life in a very short time by the clock.

"Now, it has been repeatedly demonstrated that subjective time appreciation can be hallucinated just as you can hallucinate visual or auditory sensations, in response to suggestion during hypnosis. The subject thus actually experiences the amount of subjective time that is suggested to him. So, in a sense, you have a 'special time' of your own, which you can call on as you wish. Moreover, you have an unlimited supply of it. It is the time of the dream world and of the hallucinated world, and since it is readily available, you will never have to hurry in these tests. Furthermore, it bears no relation whatever to the time of my watch, which, consequently, you will ignore.

"Knowing these things, you can now relax and take your time."

Certain suggestions other than those pertaining to specific tasks have proved useful. Among these are the following:

"As we practice these tasks, they will become easier and easier for you."

"With practice, the experiences will become more and more clear, and more and more real, so that you will actually live them."

"With each experience, you will go deeper and deeper asleep."

"The experiences will come of their own accord, promptly and effortlessly, when I give you the starting signal."

"The experiences will stop immediately, as I give you the termination signal."

Throughout the training, advantage is taken of the following:

1. The inherent tendency toward spontaneous time distortion in hallucinated activities.

2. The effort and the need on the part of the hypnotized subject to carry out suggestions, especially to finish a completed activity.
3. The fact that, at the beginning at least, familiar activities are more readily hallucinated than unfamiliar ones.
4. The fact that the interest and curiosity of the subject, and his feeling of being productive, tend to improve cooperation and performance. Advantage can be taken of this by giving him sufficient understanding of what he is doing so that he accepts and does not reject it.
5. The tendency to improve with practice.

In all training, it is of the utmost importance for the experimenter to give the subject his undivided attention when addressing him. Subjects are quick to detect the slightest deviation from this approach, and may resent highly any evidence that they themselves are not the sole object of the experimenter's interest and attention. Thus, they can often tell, by changes in his voice, when the experimenter is thinking of something else, or turning his face away, as in looking at his notes, etc., even though their eyes are closed.

It must be remembered that subjects vary widely in their capabilities as regards time distortion in hypnosis. After a few hours of training, the experimenter will have obtained a fair idea as to a given subject's ability to acquire this skill. For routine experimental work, it has been our policy to continue training with only those who are promising.

CHAPTER 7

Experimental Basis of This Report

Our first experimental work on time distortion in hypnosis was done early in 1948 (3). Three subjects were used, all of whom demonstrated the phenomenon of time distortion, and preliminary studies were done on one of these.

In the summer of 1950, a more extended study of the problem was undertaken, using 6 subjects (4). This inquiry extended over 156 experimental hours. In addition to repeating and extending experiments reported in 1948, it approached related matters such as the injection of sound signals into hallucinatory activities, mathematical mental activity, and the review and practice of previously learned material.

Since then, work has been done with six more subjects, with special emphasis upon motor learning (6), non-motor learning (5), and mathematical mental activity, association, and creative mental activity. This work has included, in addition, a certain amount of further experimentation with miscellaneous activities, metronome tasks, sound signals, and various other activities. Polygraph studies have been made with one subject.

Altogether, over 800 hours of experimental work with subjects has been done, and the author himself has undergone training as a hypnotic subject.

CHAPTER 8

Miscellaneous Activities

Any sort of activity that has meaning, to the subject, may be assigned as an experimental task. The following is a partial list of tasks assigned in this work, and will serve to give the reader a general idea of the sort of activity employed:

> Being at a certain place
> Buying various things
> Counseling
> Counting various objects
> Discussing various matters
> Doing housework
> Doing something of the subject's choice
> Dreaming
> Eating meals
> Free association
> Having one's hair cut
> Listening to music or poetry
> Picnicking
> Playing games
> Preparing talks
> Preparing meals
> Reciting poetry
> Reliving past experiences
> Sewing
> Shaving
> Studying and reviewing
> Swimming
> Thinking about various problems
> Visiting friends
> Watching games, movies, or plays
> Working at one's vocation

The following two reports are representative of those of hundreds of miscellaneous tasks which have been assigned to our subjects in the course of this work.

EXPERIMENT 1

Subject M

Task instructions: "When I give you the starting signal by saying 'Now', you'll spend a half an hour doing something you enjoy, like going on a picnic."

Allotted time: Ten seconds.

Suggested personal time: Half an hour.

Report: "My mother and sister and I were driving out in New Mexico when we decided to buy some weiners and have a picnic. The only store had no weiners, only some fat sausages, and only four of those, so we bought them and some buns and drove on to a place with big, high cliffs. Then I started to try to build a fire and found we had no matches, so I tried to light it with the lighter but it wouldn't catch. Then I twisted up a piece of newspaper and tried to poke it in the gas tank to get it saturated with gasoline, but it wouldn't poke in. About this time, a police car drove up and my sister said, "Try to act like we're not building a fire." The police said, "You having some trouble?" and I answered, "Yes, trouble building a fire." So they said, "You're just not good boy scouts. If you'd walk a couple of steps you could find some stones to strike together," and one walked back toward his car. I thought he was going to get some stones, but instead he got some matches from his car and lit a fire. I told them I was sorry we couldn't invite them to eat with us but we didn't have enough."

The seeming duration was one hour.

EXPERIMENT 2

Subject I

Task instructions: "When I give you the starting signal by saying 'Now', you're going to go swimming for 15 to 20 minutes."

Allotted time: Ten seconds.

Suggested personal time: 15 or 20 minutes.

Report: "I was on the beach, a very rocky beach, facing an extremely clear, blue sea. I ran and dived into the sea and swam under water for a minute or two. When I surfaced, I saw a raft about 200 yards ahead and swam toward it. While I was swimming, a motor boat kept zigzagging up in front of me. I finally reached the raft and lay on it for a while.

The scene was very vivid, and was notable for the blueness of the sky and water."

The seeming duration was a half hour.

COMMENT

In neither case was the experience a re-living of a previous one. The action was continuous, without omissions, and was very "real". The re-living of past experiences can, of course, be very easily produced by giving the appropriate suggestion.

Table 2 gives some of the significant data obtained in one of the earlier groups of experiments. Those not involving an allotted time were done early in the subjects' training. Those with an allotted time are examples of the subjects' better performance for this type of task. The amounts of previous training and practice varied widely.

The subjects of table 2 were selected for the experiments merely because it had been demonstrated that they were capable of experiencing, in varying degrees, the trance state. Subjects D, F, and G had had no previous experience with hypnosis; C and H had had some such experience; E, with five hours, had had the most.

There is a marked difference between subjects as regards their ability to produce the various phenomena under study. This is to be expected, and it is mentioned here in order to call attention to the fact that the amount of training required is variable within wide limits. Thus one subject may require only three hours of training while another may require twenty.

Good subjects, who have had considerable experience with time distortion, will learn to produce large amounts of hallucinatory activity in a very short allotted time (A.T.). As previously mentioned, this activity is reported as being continuous, and very "real", and proceeding at a normal or natural rate as far as the subject is concerned. Invariably, the amount of action is far in excess of what a waking individual could experience in the same allotted time. With completed activities, the seeming duration is generally appropriate. With continuous activities, the amount of action may be quite appropriate to the suggested personal time (S.P.T.), or it may be less.

Such subjects may routinely report having finished "completed" tasks, whose seeming duration is 30 to 60 minutes, in an allotted time (A.T.) of three seconds. With continuous activities, they may report a seeming duration (S.D.) of an hour or more, with an appropriate amount of activity, in a similar allotted time. One reported seeing a basketball

TABLE 2

SUB-JECT	CODE	ACTIVITY	W.T.	A.T.	S.P.T.	S.D.
C	A.T.0, B1	Walking one mile	59″			13′
C	A.T.0, B1	Watching movie short	1′35″			12′
C	A.T.0, B1	Walking to school	1′6″			20′
D	A.T.0, B1	Walking to school	1′53″			20′
D	A.T.0, B2	Painting a picture	43″			15′
E	A.T.0, B1	Listening to music (piece)	2′45″			10′
E	A.T.0, B1	Walking to school	2′17″			30′
C	A.T.+, A1	Group discussion		1′		13′
C	A.T.+, A1	Reliving		1′		1 hr. 35′
C	A.T.+, A1	Reliving		20″		15′
D	A.T.+, A1	Group discussion		1′		10′
D	A.T.+, A1	Free association		1′		15′
D	A.T.+, A1	Picnic		2′		20′
E	A.T.+, A1	Group discussion		20″		14′
E	A.T.+, A1	Shopping		20″		10′
F	A.T.+, A1	Watching races		10″		5′
C	A.T.+, B1	Considering problem		1′		20′
C	A.T.+, B1	Counseling		10″		12′
D	A.T.+, B1	Morning routine		10″		10′
D	A.T.+, B1	Making a pie		1′		15′
D	A.T.+, B2	Swimming		1′		25′
E	A.T.+, B1	Counseling		20″		10′
E	A.T.+, B1	Counseling		10″		10′
F	A.T.+, B1	Listening to music (piece)		20″		5′
F	A.T.+, B1	Watching ballet (scene)		20″		10′
F	A.T.+, B1	Problem		1′		15′
C	A.T.+, A3	Watching football game		10″	10′	10′
D	A.T.+, A3	Visiting friends		10″	10′	5–10′
F	A.T.+, A3	Watching races		10″	10′	10′
F	A.T.+, A3	Swimming		10″	10′	8′
F	A.T.+, A3	Dancing		10″	10′	10′
C	A.T.+, B3	Considering a decision		30″	1 hr.	1 hr.

game in an allotted time of one second. Another counted 9200 BB shot, one by one, in five seconds. He was seated, in a bathing suit, alongside a swimming pool and threw the shot into a bucket as he counted them. After counting each 2000, he would swim the length of the pool. As his fingers were moist, he had some difficulty handling the shot, as they are small. The demonstrated rate was 72 per minute. Other subjects have taken long walks, been on "dates" or at dances or picnics, watched games, done shopping, talked with friends, prepared lectures, relived former experiences, etc., in an allotted time of 10 seconds. Such activities, in the waking state, would take from half an hour to several hours.

An analysis of a large number of tasks involving miscellaneous activities permits the following statements to be made concerning them.

Experiential time

If we simply assign a prolonged, completed activity to a subject and ask him to let us know when he has finished it, we shall find the following to be true:

    a. He will complete the activity.
    b. It will appear to proceed at the usual rate.
    c. It will probably take less than three minutes by world time.
    d. It will seem, to the subject, to take much longer.

In other words, there will be definite time distortion even though the suggestion made no stipulation whatever concerning time.

These relations are shown in an analysis of 55 tasks in which the activity was a completed one, and in which there was no allotted time (A.T.) or suggested personal time (S.P.T.):

World time
    Average... 127 secs.
    Maximum....................................... 270 secs.
    Minimum....................................... 35 secs.

S.D.
    Average... 17 min.
    Maximum....................................... 45 min.
    Minimum....................................... 3 min.

S.D. was invariably longer than W.T.

It is thus seen that, in hallucinatory activity in hypnosis, there is apparently an inherent tendency for time distortion to occur.

Another basic consideration is the fact that the subject will try his best to carry out whatever is suggested—to "obey orders" in other words. Thus if, with a given activity, we use an allotted time and gradually decrease this in repeated tasks, assuring the subject that he will not have to hurry and will have plenty of time, he will learn somehow to adjust his hallucinated action to the short world time interval. He will "fit it in", so to speak. Yet he will continue to complete the assignment without hurrying, it will appear to be real in every way, and the experiential time will be appropriate. Use is made of this in training subjects, and it is of considerable importance for this reason.

A little reflection will reveal that in assigning a completed activity we not only assign a definite amount of action, but also, in effect, an appropriate amount of experiential time. This is especially true if we tell the subject not to hurry. The reason for this, of course, is that the awareness of action or change is invariably accompanied by a sense of the passage of time.

On the other hand, time sense itself may be prolonged without the awareness of an equivalent amount of action. This is seen in the dream, when there is often a relative poverty of action. It is also true in those hypnotically induced hallucinations where, on occasions generally involving a suggested personal time (S.P.T.), the amount of activity, though large, is still much less than would be expected when one considers the seeming duration (S.D.).

We can see from the above that, in hypnotically induced hallucinations, the experiential time is influenced by some inherent factor, and by the assigned activity itself.

A third consideration, and a most effective one, is the direct suggestion of a subjective time interval—the use of a suggested personal time (S.P.T.).

Amount of action

Where a continuous activity is used, and there is no suggested personal time (S.P.T.), the accomplishment depends upon the rate at which the subject chooses to carry out his hallucinated action and the allotted time (A.T.) or world time (W.T.).

On the other hand, where a continuous activity is used and a suggested personal time (S.P.T.) given, the subject will strive to fill up his suggested interval with action. Most of our counting experiments are of this type and are indeed remarkable.

With a completed activity, the most important factor determining the amount of action is, of course, the assignment itself. Within undetermined limits, a proficient subject will complete activities as requested.

SUMMARY

The essential points in the above discussion of the relation between type of activity, S.P.T., amount of activity, and S.D. are recapitulated below:

I. Continuous activity.
   a. Without S.P.T.
      Amount of action depends upon subject's chosen speed of hallucinatory action, and upon A.T. or W.T.
      S.D. will be appropriate to the action.
   b. With S.P.T.
      Amount of action will be consistent with S.P.T. where the subject is proficient.
      S.D. will equal S.P.T.
II. Completed activity.
   a. Without S.P.T.
      Amount of action is determined by the suggested activity.
      S.D. is appropriate to the suggested activity.
   b. With S.P.T.
      Amount of action is determined by the suggested activity.
      S.D. equals S.P.T.

It is understood, of course, that the subject has had enough training to have become proficient. Thus, in a sense, the above statements apply to the "ideal" subject. The commonest short-coming is an inability fully to accept a suggested personal time (S.P.T.).

It is clear from the above that hallucinated action and subjective time are, to a certain degree, inter-related.

Time distortion, as effected in these experiments, is accompanied by a marked increase in the ratio S.D./W.T. It is usually accompanied by an appropriate increase in hallucinated activity. In order to produce these results, then, the following conditions should be fulfilled:

For a continuous activity:
   A familiar activity.
   S.P.T.—long.
   A.T.—short.
For a completed activity:
   A familiar activity the completion of which requires a relatively long period of time.
   S.P.T.—not of primary importance. If used, it should be appropriate.
   A.T.—short.
In general:
   Subjects often find that the suggestion, "Please don't hurry, you'll have plenty of time," reassures them and helps them to relax.

CHAPTER 9

Counting

By far the most dramatic results were those obtained in the counting experiments. These were usually run as continuous activities with a short allotted time (A.T.) and a moderately long suggested personal time (S.P.T.). In a few instances, however, the suggestion was put in the completed form by saying, "Since you can easily count 30 in a minute, you will have no difficulty counting at least 300 in ten minutes. Please take your time and don't hurry." This was generally done during training, in an attempt to utilize the performance-increasing value of the completed activity. In still others, it was suggested to the subject that he count a definite number of objects.

Sometimes the subject was given a "preview" of his surroundings in the following manner:

"You now see several large bags of gum drops on a table. Please tell me what you see."

Then, after a brief description by the subject, "Stay there now, and listen to me."

The activity suggestion was then given.

It is by no means necessary to use a "preview", and in the later experiments it was omitted, the instructions being like those in experiment 4. This is in keeping with our policy of avoiding concurrent reporting.

Table 3 shows the results of some of the earlier counting experiments. The subjects belong to the same group as those whose performances are tabulated in table 2.

It will be noted that the count, although much greater than the product (D.R.)(W.T.), is almost invariably less than (D.R.)(S.D.). Sometimes the subjects had no explanation for this. At other times they ascribed the discrepancy to the fact that part of the time was occupied otherwise than by counting.

The following individual experiments will give the reader a far better idea of this type of task than any general discussion could possibly provide. The letter E stands for experimenter, S for subject.

TABLE 3

SUB-JECT	CODE	COUNTING	A.T.	S.P.T.	S.D.	COUNT	D.R.	D.R. × S.D.
A	A.T.+, A3	Flowers	10″	10′	8′	140		
A	A.T.+, A3	Flowers	10″	10′	7′	41	48	336
A	A.T.+, A3	Flowers	10″	10′	10′	35	42	420
A	A.T.+, B3	Pennies (50)†	10″	10′	3′	28	19	57
A	A.T.+, A3	Potatoes	10″	10′	5′	165	60	300
A	A.T.+, A3	Candies	10″	10′	5′	140	60	300
A	A.T.+, A3	Candies	10″	10′	8′	402	60	480
A	A.T.+, A3	Candies	10″	10′	3′	75	60	180
C	A.T.+, B3	Flowers (150)†	10″	10′*	10′	145		
C	A.T.+, B3	Pearls (200)†	10″	10′	10′	100		
C	A.T.+, A3	Candies	10″	10′	10′	127		
C	A.T.+, A3	Candies	10″	10′	8′	49		
C	A.T.+, A3	Candies	10″	10′	10′	127		
E	A.T.+, A3	Flowers	20″	20′*	20′	115	54	1080
E	A.T.+, A3	Flowers	20″	20′*	20′	40	35	700
E	A.T.+, A3	Strawberries	20″	60′*	50′	600		
E	A.T.+, A3	Tomatoes	20″	60′*	40′	225		
E	A.T.+, A3	Bullets	10″	10′*	10′	546	54	540
E	A.T.+, A3	Flowers	10″	15′*	15′	973	60	900
E	A.T.+, A3	Cookies	10″	20′*	23′	1003	60	1380
F	A.T.+, A3	Nuts	20″	20′*	20′	400	66	1320
F	A.T.+, B3	Candies (200)†	10″	10′*	60′	2500	72	4320
F	A.T.+, A3	Flowers	10″	10′*	10′	60		

* Time suggestion was preceded by the phrase "at least".
† Subject to count at least this number.

EXPERIMENT 1

Subject B

E. You're back on the farm, and are going to churn some butter. Tell me what you see.

S. (Subject described the scene in some detail. She was sitting on the back porch, with a crockery churn half full of milk. She mentioned the paddle with the "crosspiece" on it, and the hole in the top of the churn, through which the paddle passes.)

E. Now just stay there for a while, and listen carefully. You're going to churn that milk, and it's going to take you ten minutes, which will be plenty of time. While churning, you're going to count the strokes. I shall give you a signal to start, and another signal, at the end of ten minutes, to stop. Here comes the signal—"Start".[1]

[1] In the early experiments, the word "start" was used as the starting signal instead of "now".

(Three seconds later)

E. Now stop. The ten minutes are up. Now make your mind a blank. Your mind is a blank. Now tell me about it. Tell me what you did, how high you counted, and how long you were churning.

S. (She reported that she counted 114 strokes, and churned for ten minutes. Everything was very real to her. The churning became more difficult toward the end as the butter formed, and this slowed things down. She heard the churning, and had plenty of time. At the "stop" signal the entire scene faded from view.)

E. Show me, by counting out loud, how you counted the strokes.

S. (She counted to 60 in one minute, adding that toward the end the strokes became slower because of the increased resistance from the butter.)

E. I'm going to wake you up by counting to ten. You will remember all about this experience and tell me about it.

S. (On waking she is again asked to give a report. Her story is similar to the above, including the number of strokes counted, the time estimate, and the demonstrated rate.)

In this example, then, the world time (W.T.) and the allotted time (A.T.) was three seconds, the suggested personal time (S.P.T.) 10 minutes, the seeming duration (S.D.) 10 minutes, and the demonstrated rate (D.R.) 60 strokes per minute.

The product of the demonstrated rate times the seeming duration (D.R.)(S.D.) is 600. Yet the subject insists that she took only 114 strokes, that she counted each stroke individually, and that she was occupied for the full ten minutes. When asked, post-hypnotically, about the discrepancy, she had no explanation to offer.

EXPERIMENT 2

Subject G

E. What would you like to do now?

S. My husband molds bullets for his gun. I could be counting them as he makes them.

E. For how long do you want to do this?

S. For ten minutes.

E. When I give you the starting signal by saying "Now", you're going to spend at least ten minutes of your special time counting bullets as your husband makes them. If the sound signal is given, you will be aware of it. Here comes the starting signal—"Now".

(The pitch instrument was sounded from the fourth to the seventh second.)

(Ten seconds later)

E. Now make your mind a blank. Your mind is now a blank. Now tell me about it.

S. It was at a molding party of the club. There was quite a crowd there. I counted for maybe six minutes and ran out of bullets, so I waited for more. I didn't count the full ten minutes. While I was counting them this other boy walked up—he was talking and waving his arms. The pot of lead tipped over. It burned his foot rather badly. I got up but then sat down again and continued counting. The others were running all over the place. The remainder of the lead we put back on the stove. I counted 493. That's when I stopped and waited. Then later I got up to 546.

E. Did you hurry?

S. I didn't hurry too much as I was counting, but I kept busy.

E. Was it real?

S. Yes.

E. When I give you the signal to start, please show me, by counting aloud, how you counted the bullets. Now.

S. (Subject counted at a rate of 54 per minute.)

E. Were you aware of the sound signal?

S. When they spilt the lead it sizzled a lot.

E. How long was the sizzling?

S. It seemed like three or four minutes.

(This interpolation of the sound signal into the hallucinated activity will be discussed later.)

EXPERIMENT 3

Subject G

E. What would you like to do now?

S. To package some cookies. I used to do this.

E. For how long?

S. Twenty minutes.

E. When I give you the starting signal by saying "now", you're going to spend at least twenty minutes of your special time packaging cookies. As you do this, you'll count them. If the sound signal is given, you will be aware of it. Here comes the starting signal—"Now".

(The pitch instrument was sounded from the fifth to the eighth second.)

(Ten seconds later)

E. Now make your mind a blank. Your mind is now a blank. Now tell me about it, please.

S. I was down in the basement. There were work tables. I was counting. I counted them as I put them in the smaller sacks. I counted 1003. That was all I got. In the middle the telephone outside rang on and on. Just after that there was so much cookie dust all over that I started to sneeze. I sneezed ten or twelve times. I just couldn't stop. I dropped one package. I didn't answer the phone.

E. When I give you the signal to start, please show me, by counting aloud, how you counted the cookies. Now.

S. (Subject counted at a rate of sixty per minute.)

E. How long did the telephone ring?

S. It must have been five or six minutes. No one answered it outside.

EXPERIMENT 4

Subject I

Task instructions: "When I give you the starting signal by saying 'Now', you will find yourself seated at a table. On the table will be a large box of pennies. You will take the pennies from the box, one at a time, and place them on the table, counting them as you do so. You will do this for ten minutes."

Suggested personal time: In the first seven tasks, this was kept constant. In the last four, it was varied.

Allotted time: In the first seven tasks, this was varied. In the last four, it was kept constant.

Comment

Reducing the allotted time to 5 seconds in task 2 is accompanied by a lowering of the count and of the seeming duration. Further reduction

TABLE 4
Counting pennies

TASK	S.P.T.	A.T.	COUNT	S.D. OF INTERVAL BETWEEN SIGNALS	S.D. OF COUNTING	D.R.
1	10′	10″	419	10′	10′	60/min.
2	10′	5″	390	8′	8′	66/min.
3	10′	3″	401	10′	10′	60/min.
4	10′	1″	312	6′	6′	72/min.
5	10′	1″	293	4′	4′	66/min.
6	10′	1″	372	8′	8′	72/min.
7	10′	1″	402	10′	10′	66/min.
8	10′	10″	612	12′	10′	66/min.
9	5′	10″	311	8′	5′	60/min.
10	20′	10″	1147	20′	20′	60/min.
11	1′	10″	69	10′	1′	66/min.

to 3 seconds in task 3 does not show this effect, as the subject has adjusted to the shortened allotted time. In tasks 4 and 5, with an allotted time of one second, we again see the same effect as in task 2, but full recovery has been made in task 7.

Having adjusted to an allotted time of one second, it is interesting to note that in task 8, with an allotted time of 10 seconds, the count is increased. The subject reported that he "counted for the first ten minutes and then waited for the termination signal. I just sat there and ran my hands through the pile of coins, spreading them over the table." In tasks 9 and 11, he likewise finished his five minutes and one minute counting, respectively, and then sat waiting for the termination signal.

These tasks show that, with a constant suggested personal time, the count varies with the allotted time, until an adjustment is made as in task 7. When the allotted time is constant, the count varies with the suggested personal time.

Subjects undoubtedly have an idea how many objects they ordinarily would count in the suggested personal time and tend to approach that figure.

CHAPTER 10

Sound Signals

The idea of exploring hallucinatory activities by means of injected sound signals was suggested to us by Dr. J. B. Rhine (14).

In one group of tests the subjects were told to take a familiar walk—from house to school. No allotted time (A.T.), or suggested personal time (S.P.T.), was used. Upon finishing, the subject said "Now". A single short sound signal, produced by striking a damped glass with a metal knife, was employed at various intervals from the start. The subject was then asked to estimate, at the end of the test, the personal time of the entire experience and the approximate location of the sound signal. The latter they usually did by considering where, in their walk, they were when they heard the signal. Figure 1 shows the relation of the signal to world and experiential times.

In other cases a pitch instrument was sounded for a known length of time during an activity with an allotted time. The subject was later asked to estimate its duration. Some of the results are shown in table 6.

The subjects, even though forewarned, were not always aware of the sound signal, and when they were, it was experienced in various forms.

Striking the glass, to some subjects, sounded exactly as it does normally, and did not take on any significance in the hypnotic scene. More often, however, it was heard as a somewhat similar sound, such as a tumbler dropping on the floor, ice striking the side of the pitcher, an object falling on a hard surface, etc. Sometimes, however, the actual sound signal acquired an entirely different significance, e.g. the sizzling of the lead and the ringing of the telephone noted above.

Since the subject had been led to expect a sound signal, he quite possibly anticipated it and included appropriate "properties" in his hallucination. Thus, in three successive counseling scenes, glass was present either as a tumbler or a pitcher.

Even so, there is much food for thought here, for an object must fall before it can strike the floor and make a noise, and there must be some

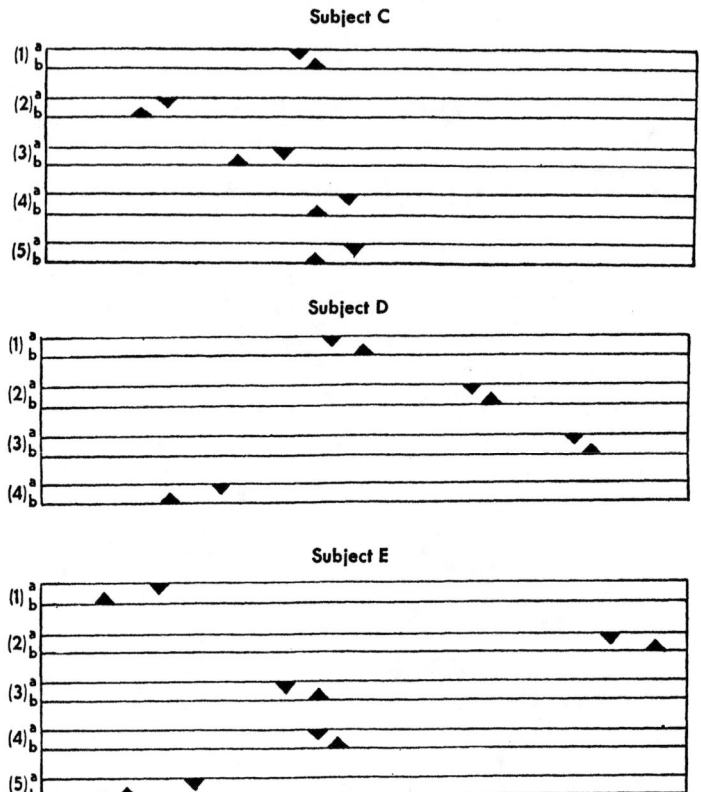

Fig. 1. Based on the data shown in table 5. The pairs of lines represent the world time interval (a), and the personal time interval (b), for a given test. The markers show where the sound signal actually occurred in relation to the world time interval (on lines a), and its location in the personal time interval (on lines b), as determined by asking the subject how long it seemed from the beginning of the activity to the signal. Note that the subject locates the signals with fair accuracy.

cause for the fall. Somehow or other, all this is arranged in a most skillful way. Interestingly enough, to one subject the sound signal came just as he struck a pole with a stick. After telling about it, he added, "I had anticipated hitting the pole, for I saw it in the distance." It may be that there is a definite lag between the communication of the signal to the brain and its entry into the hallucinated world as an appropriate part of the picture.

Similarly with the pitch instrument, at times it was unchanged, but more often it was altered.

TABLE 5

| | WORLD TIME (SEC.) | | SEEMING DURATION (MIN.) | |
	Signal	Total	Signal	Total
Subject C				
(1)	60	155	5	12
(2)	20	105	1.5	10
(3)	60	164	3.5	12
(4)	90	192	5	12
(5)	120	252	5	12
Subject D				
(1)	60	133	10	20
(2)	90	135	14	20
(3)	110	133	17	20
(4)	30	107	4	20
Subject E				
(1)	30	163	3	30
(2)	120	137	28.5	30
(3)	60	159	13	30
(4)	90	210	17	37
(5)	46	196	4	30

TABLE 6

| SUBJECT | ACTIVITY | CODE | A.T. | S.P.T. | S.D. | SOUND SIGNAL | | |
						Time (sec.)	Appearance form	Est. duration
E	Baking cake	A.T.+, B3	15″	15′	10′	5th–10th	Auto horn stuck	3 or 4′
E	Mowing lawn	A.T.+, A3	10″	10′	10′	3rd– 5th	Squeaking	2′
E	Counting bullets	A.T.+, A3	10″	10′	10′	4th– 7th	Sizzling lead	3 or 4′
E	Picking flowers	A.T.+, A3	10″	15′	15′	5th– 8th	Bird singing	5′
E	Embroidering	A.T.+, A3	10″	15′	15′	4th– 7th	Radio static	3 or 4′
E	Counting cookies	A.T.+, A3	10″	20′	23′	5th– 8th	Telephone ring	5 or 6′
F	Watching basketball	A.T.+, A3	10″	10′	5′	5th– 6th	"Funny noise"	1′
F	Picnic	A.T.+, A1	20″		20′	10th–15th	"Like a train"	"Quite a while"

The presence in our group of two musicians, one with "absolute pitch", gave us the opportunity of determining whether a sound, coming into the hallucinated world of altered time sense, would itself be altered in tone, i.e., lowered, by virtue of the new time relations (8). The answer apparently depends upon the degree to which the sound is disguised. In hallucinations where it was heard as a horn and an air-raid "all clear", the pitch was recognized as C. Usually, however, there was little resemblance to the original, the pitch instrument being heard variously as a bird, a fan, a squeaky lawn-mower, the buzzing of a crowd of people, etc.

Of considerable significance is the fact that almost always the duration of the sound seemed much longer than it actually was. This is what we would expect in the presence of time distortion and, in a way, confirms the reports of the subjects. Here too we have the awareness of a physical phenomenon during time distortion, and the event seems to be slowed. Compare this with reports from persons following a narrow escape, who may say that world events appeared to be in "slow motion".

Not always was the intruder welcome, for on several occasions the hallucination was completely destroyed. On others the subject would become "nervous", irritated, or apprehensive.

In fact, one subject reported that in subsequent walks, whenever he passed the spot at which he had previously been "jolted" by the sound signal, he had a sense of impending trouble. Here, apparently, we have an instance of conditioning to a hallucinated environment. This is evidence of the subjective reality of the experience.

We have, on a few occasions, injected brief sounds into continuous counting activities in which an allotted time was used, asking the subject to note the number of the object that he is handling when he hears the signal. Results sometimes check closely, but at other times they do not. This inconsistency is undoubtedly related to the mechanism whereby the subject adapts his experience to an allotted time, and is most obscure.

CHAPTER 11

Metronome

The first experiment in time distortion was undertaken in order to determine whether, in the hypnotized subject, the seeming duration of the time interval between two sounds can be prolonged by means of direct suggestion in the trance state. A "good" subject, entirely ignorant of the nature of the experiment, was placed in a moderately deep trance state by means of suggestions of sleep. After induction had been accomplished, a metronome was started, the rate being one stroke per second. The subject was told that the sounds she heard were being produced by a metronome, and that the rate was one stroke per second. The experimenter then told her that he was going to slow down the metronome gradually, and that she was to listen carefully as he did so. When, in her opinion, the metronome had been slowed down till its rate was only one stroke per *minute*, she was to notify the experimenter by saying, "Now".

Having given these instructions, the experimenter, *while the metronome continued to strike at a constant rate of one stroke per second*, said, "It's going slower and slower—slower and slower—slower and slower, etc." These suggestions were spaced at intervals of from five to 15 seconds.

After a minute or so, the subject said, "Now". When asked how fast the metronome was going, she replied, "About one stroke per minute." The metronome was then stopped, and the subject was waked, whereupon she confirmed the report given in the trance state.

It is obvious from the above that, if the subject's report is a true description of her experience, towards the end of the experiment the interval between two successive metronome strokes, actually one second in length as "measured" by the clock, seemed to her to be about one minute. In other words, the interval was similar to that which she generally experiences between two events that are one minute apart. The same interval *seemed* to the *experimenter* to be about one second. Thus, as a result of suggestion in the trance state, the subject had finally experienced a series of intervals, each with a seeming duration of about a minute, between the metronome strokes. On the other hand, the *experimenter* experienced intervals that seemed to be of about a second each, between the *same* strokes. Since interval constitutes one form of *experiential time*, we can say that this experiment suggests that experiential time was actually "given" to the hypnotized subject by means of suggestion. This marked difference between the seeming duration of an interval and its clock reading constitutes time distortion.

It is seen in the above experiment that the experiencing by the subject of each interval, the seeming duration of which was, to her, one minute, took place between two "physical" events (two successive metronome strokes) spaced at an interval of world time (one second) that was determined by the experimenter and was unknown to the subject.

Using the terminology presented in Chapter 3, these results may be tabulated as follows:

> Task—to experience a sense of duration of 1 minute
> Suggested personal time—1 minute
> Seeming duration (to subject)—1 minute
> Allotted time—1 second
> World time—1 second

In the second experiment, the subject was again told that the metronome would be slowed to one stroke per minute. She was to indicate this occurrence by saying, "Now", as she had done previously. After she had complied she was told that she would be given a signal (tap on the forearm) at which time she would start to review in her "mind's eye" some of her school days during the fifth grade, seeing in her imagination the school, the teacher, and her companions. She would do this for ten *minutes*—that is, ten strokes of the metronome—at the end of which time she would be notified to stop.

The metronome was stopped after ten beats—ten *seconds*, world time—and the subject was waked up. On questioning, the following significant experiences were recounted:

1. The metronome was most certainly "slowed down".
2. A good 10 minutes had elapsed between signals.
3. She had "lots of time", and saw clearly the school and her classmates.
4. She expressed great surprise when told that the metronome had not changed rate, and that actually her experience had taken only ten seconds.

Here again, time sense was altered, to a predetermined degree, by the experimenter. In addition, the subject reported an amount of experience that was more nearly commensurate with the subjective time involved than with the world time. *This activity seemed to proceed at a normal or natural rate as far as she was concerned.*

The data on this experiment are:

> Task—visiting her school
> Suggested personal time—10 minutes
> Seeming duration (to subject)—10 minutes
> Allotted time—10 seconds
> World time—10 seconds

The above experiments indicate that the experience of duration itself may be altered by suggestion in the trance state, and that large amounts of hallucinatory experience, proceeding at a normal rate as far as the subject is concerned, may be had in very brief periods of clock time.

TRAINING AND FURTHER EXPERIMENTAL REPORTS

In training a subject for metronome experiments, he is put into the trance state and then the metronome is started, the rate being one stroke per second. The subject is told that the sounds are being produced by a metronome, that the rate is one stroke per second, and that he is to listen to it carefully. He is then told that the experimenter is going to slow it down gradually, and that when its rate has decreased to one stroke per minute, he (the subject) is to notify the experimenter by saying "Now".

The metronome is actually allowed to continue at its original rate, but the experimenter says, from time to time, "It's going slower and slower—slower and slower—slower and slower," etc. These suggestions are spaced at intervals of from five to 15 seconds.

Some subjects are unable to accept such suggestions and will report either no slowing, or only slight slowing. Other subjects will accept them fully and, after a varying length of time, will say, "Now". The instrument is then stopped, and the subject is asked for his report, which will be to the effect that the metronome actually slowed down to one stroke per minute.

The metronome is again started, the rate being one stroke per second. The subject is told to listen to it for a while, and he is told its true rate. The following suggestion is then given: "When I give you the starting signal, by saying 'Now', you will start counting the metronome strokes, each of which you will hear. As you listen and count, the metronome will go slower and slower. When, in your opinion, its rate has slowed down to one stroke every 20 seconds, you will let me know by saying 'Now'." (The counting is, of course, purely hallucinated counting. The subject actually remains silent and motionless.) At the termination signal, the metronome is stopped. Proficient subjects will report the same count as the experimenter.

The above experiment may be varied by including, in the task instructions, the expression, "In between strokes, you will engage in any sort of hallucinatory activity that you wish." In such a case, good subjects will have a variety of experiences in the intervals.

The criteria for success in the metronome tasks are that the subject's count of the metronome strokes be the same as the experimenter's, and that the subject report a slowing of the metronome to the stipulated rate.

Metronome training was given to six subjects and succeeded in three.

CHAPTER 12

Review and Practice

A few pilot experiments were run in an effort to learn whether our subjects could review for a history examination in distorted time. The results were inconclusive, but it led one of them, a professional violinist, to attempt to review certain pieces and to practice these while in a self-induced trance, using her "special time" for this purpose. Her own account of the procedure follows.

"I put myself into a trance and then practiced in several different ways. I might see the music before me and mark the spots that needed extra practice. I would then play the different spots over and over until I got them—which helped my finger memory because I was actually playing in the trance." (This was hallucinated activity only. In other words, she was "actually playing" only in the hallucinated world and not in the physical world.)

"I did 'passage practice'—picking hard passages and playing them in several ways to facilitate speed and accuracy."

"Then I went through the whole composition for continuity. In doing this in 'special time' I seemed to get an immediate grasp of the composition as a whole."

Thus she was able to practice and review long pieces over and over in very brief world time periods, and she found that not only did her memory improve strikingly, but also her technical performance. This remarkable result is attested to by her husband, himself a musician. In other words, she felt that hallucinated practice of these pieces, learned years ago, improved her subsequent performance.

It is impossible at present to evaluate these reports which, if confirmed, carry important implications for facilitation of the learning process. They suggest at least two possibilities for making use of distorted time in the hypnotized subject.

The first is that the memorizing of new material might be speeded up by hallucinating the frequent repetition, either in visual or auditory form, of whatever is to be learned. The second, of course, is that halluci-

63

nated practice and review be used to aid in the acquiring of new motor skills.

Reports on inquiry into these two possibilities will be presented in subsequent chapters.

CHAPTER 13

Coincidental Happenings

Not infrequently certain fortuitous and sometimes unwelcome things occurred and were reported. They are listed here because they so convincingly bespeak the reality of these experiences, all of which occurred during time distortion.

While rowing a boat, the subject lost an oarlock.

While picking up shells, he stepped on a jelly-fish.

While getting out of the way of an automobile, he tripped over the curb.

"Mother helped me on with my coat. It wouldn't button. Dad buttoned the vest."

In changing a tire, he found only 3 lugs in place. Later he found the fourth one in the hub-cap.

"I hurried to get past a hayfield which was irritating my nose."

In changing electric light bulbs, the one he threw into the scrapbasket broke.

While drilling, the man next to him "passed out" from heat prostration.

Asked to sing a hymn in church, "I stood on the platform and announced to the Baptists that I was going to sing a Jewish chant. I sang it all the way through." (In an allotted time of 10 seconds.)

While burning trash, he watched the match burn down, after striking it on his pants.

"I shaved but I didn't wash my face afterwards. I didn't have authority to do that." (Suggestion "You're going to shave." A.T. 10 seconds.)

"The barn door stuck because it had been raining."

"While getting shaved, the barber spent so much time talking to the other barber that the lather began to set."

While pulling up and counting iris, "The reason it took so long was because I had to get the dirt off them."

While watching a football game, his attention was drawn away from the play by a fight in the stands.

In counting potatoes, as he removed them from a basket and placed them in a sack, some fell back into the basket and hit the rim. "I had to count them over again."

While counting candies as he removed them from a box, "There was a strawberry cream that had been mashed and cracked and had run a little bit. What to do with it passed through my mind."

In counting gum-drops, he noticed that some were stuck together. "I pulled out the whole bunch and broke them off and put them in separate piles."

While picking berries, the carton got so full that they kept falling out.

While riding the waves during a swim, she hit the bottom.

While washing the baby, she spilled all the water.

In making sandwiches, she cut her finger with the knife, and it bled.

In counting chickens, she noticed that one had started sprouting wing feathers, and one was sick.

In playing truth and consequences, "They blindfolded me and a fellow kissed me and embarrassed me."

"The Victrola started slowly. I had to wind it again."

While roller-skating, she fell down.

While crocheting, the thread broke.

In buying shoes, she tried on four pairs first.

A student who came for counseling said, "I want you to know that I'm not here because I'm crazy."

While counting chickens, the first "lousy chicken" defecated in his hand. Asked what he then did, he replied, "I wiped it off on the second chicken."

A subject "got bored" while reviewing a college course.

At a picnic, a snake frightened the subject.

While busy sewing, "I was interrupted by someone coming to the door."

In doing mathematical problems, "I had to go over them again sometimes."

"While walking, I met my schoolteacher. She stopped and talked about 3 minutes."

A teacher who was checking a subject's results made her nervous because she "talked so much".

While bowling, she fell down and "skinned" her knee.

While dancing, the heel broke on one of the subject's shoes. "It embarrassed me," she said.

While in swimming, she broke the clasp on her bathing suit.

One subject, in picking flowers, reported that she had so many in her arms that they interfered with the task, adding, "You can't pick with flowers in your face."

While sewing, a subject had trouble with the machine. "It kept turning around."

COMMENT

Some subjects report such happenings far more frequently than do others. Those listed above were taken from the records of nine subjects.

CHAPTER 14

Special Inquiry

In this section, certain aspects of hallucinatory experience under conditions of time distortion in hypnosis will be discussed. Although we present this material at this point, it is to be understood that it is based upon the entire body of experimental work upon which this treatise is founded.

FALSIFICATION

As mentioned elsewhere, there is a marked tendency for readers to discount our subjects' reports, on the assumption that they represent falsification or elaboration. This is very understandable, and the question that it raises is, of course, of paramount importance. We have already pointed out that time distortion in the nocturnal dream is a very common experience, and therefore is accepted as a fact. Unfortunately, the number of persons who have experienced time distortion in hypnosis, and the related phenomena, is at present extremely small. Hence the critical reader, not having had the experience, demands what he calls "objective" evidence in this latter case, even though he readily accepts reports concerning dreams without this. In fact, it is at present impossible to demonstrate, "objectively", another person's experience.

There are, however, methods of approach which might support or controvert the assumption that the subjects are telling the truth as they know it. Among these are the following:

1. The demonstration of the ability of the subject to "utilize" his distorted time by performing simple mathematical operations, or coding problems not involving mathematics. At present, we have no evidence that this can be done. This is discussed in Chapter 20.
2. The demonstration of physiological changes appropriate to alleged emotional experiences. This has been done in trance state

studies without using time distortion. With time distortion, it has not been attempted, but success would appear unlikely because the experience proceeds at such a rapid rate relative to world time that gross physiological changes would not be expected. Possible exceptions would be electromyographic and electroencephalographic studies.

3. Recall of details of forgotten experiences on reliving them in distorted time. We have done this with a few subjects, with success. One subject relived her 4th birthday, and many of the details were found to be accurate when checked by her mother. The subject was in her thirties at the time of the experiment. Another subject relived rehearsals of a play staged 10 years previously, and recovered a good deal of lost material. A third, a pianist, apparently recovered lost skill in the performance of a piano piece learned years before, by hallucinatory practice. There have been other similar cases. In each instance, the recall occurred during experience in distorted time.

4. "Utilization of distorted time to facilitate creative mental activity. This is discussed in Chapter 17.

5. "Utilization" of distorted time to facilitate the learning process. This is discussed in Chapters 18 and 19.

6. Therapeutic results from the employment of time distortion in hypnosis for the reliving of past experiences.

7. The experiencing of the sort of phenomenon under discussion by the experimenter himself.

8. The use of the polygraph. (*See page 120.*)

Listed below are certain less conclusive considerations, which seem to indicate that the subjects are telling the truth as they know it.

1. The intuition of the experimenter who has listened to many reports, questioned many subjects, and observed their manner of answering.

2. The inherent honesty of the subjects, and their scientific interest.

3. The insistence, by the subjects, that the reporting was an entirely different event from the hallucinatory experience.

4. The subjects' often bitter resentment at being suspected of falsification. Several subjects, after repeated cross-examination, threatened to quit.

5. The direction of questions directly to the unconscious, a technique used by Erickson.
6. The results of "injecting" sound signals into hallucinated activities where no allotted time was used.
7. The spontaneous expression by the subject of emotion during reporting, in some instances, and his subsequent amazement at learning the true time relations involved.
8. The "incidental happenings" with which our reports are replete.
9. The hearing of long pieces of music, in very short periods of world time, by trained musicians. A piece of music is a pattern, extended in experiential time, and these reports support the allegations of other subjects to the effect that their experiences have continuity.
10. Apparent practice effects, noted by a second musician during actual performance, after purely hallucinated practice in distorted time.
11. The following isolated incidents furnish evidence of the truth of the subjects' reports:
    a) The carrying out of advice received from hallucinated friends (Page 72).
    b) An instance of conditioning to an hallucinated environment (Page 58).
    c) A case of synchronized hallucinated and actual motor activity (Page 102).

Let us now consider the hypothesis that our subjects are telling the truth as they know it, but that their reports are based on what we shall term "false memories". Such "memories" are "false" because they do not represent an actual previous event.

Normally, in the process of recall, a person during a time interval t_3–t_4 has an experience, termed a memory, which is believed by him to represent a previous experience had by him during an earlier interval t_1–t_2. Let us assume that an individual experiences recall as above defined and let us refer to it as "case 1".

Now, it is conceivable that, under certain conditions, a person might, during an interval t_3–t_4, have an experience that has, as far as he is concerned, all the marks of a memory, but which actually is *not* a representation of an experience during any previous interval t_1–t_2. Let us assume that an individual has such an experience, and let us refer to it as "case 2". Such recall would then be based on a "false memory" as above defined.

It is obvious that in a "case 1" type of situation, provided that the experience during t_1–t_2 occurred in the "public world", its factuality can often be established. On the other hand, where the earlier experience was an event that did not occur in the "public world", as in the case of a dream, it is much more difficult to prove that it took place. The alleged experiences of our subjects during the t_1–t_2 intervals resemble dreams in this regard.

It is therefore important to consider the possibility that our subjects' experiences during the t_3–t_4 intervals are akin to those in the "case 2" type of experience and therefore do not actually represent any earlier event. If such be the case, our subjects are not experiencing true recall, as defined at the beginning of this discussion.

It is our opinion that our subjects actually fall into the "case 1" group. The following considerations are cited in support of this opinion:

1. The findings reported in Chapters 17 and 19 concerning creative mental activity and non-motor learning.
2. The fact that sound signals, given at time t_1, or during an interval t_1–t_2, are mentioned in the reports as an integral part of the alleged hallucinatory experiences. Incidentally, such "public world" sounds have often been reported to appear in nocturnal dreams.

REALNESS

In the accomplished subject the hallucinations possess a high degree of "realness", which is fairly consistent. At times, however, reports will mention a lack of clearness in the imagery. Such instances are, on the whole, infrequent. Often, however, the definition and clarity will be confined to those things which occupy the immediate attention, the background remaining vague.

As training develops the ability to hallucinate, so also it aids in the production of scenes that are real and true to life. Thus, with practice, there comes an increase in detail and in color. To encourage this, we daily gave our subjects the following suggestion—"In this trance any scenes you see will be very clear and any experiences you have will be very real, so that you will actually live them."

One very striking evidence of the realness of the activities is the frequent reporting of accidental or coincidental happenings. For instance, the subject who is crocheting breaks her thread, and later cuts her finger while making sandwiches or spills the water in which she is bathing her child. Another one, asked to burn some rubbish, strikes the match on his pants and watches it as it burns, or, while walking past a hayfield, begins to sneeze. The chalk that the angry teacher throws strikes the blackboard and breaks, and the little boy, whose ears stand out so far, scratches his head as he strives to find the answer to his problem. Such telltale details were frequently mentioned, and a partial list of them is given elsewhere.

It was not uncommon for the subjects to say how much they enjoyed an activity and how much they regretted its termination. At other times they would get tired or become bored. In one case, a subject who had been waked was telling about an activity in which he seemed to be quite young. After telling how rough the ground was over which he had been dragging a bushel basket of apples, he asked, "Did I breathe hard?" When answered in the negative he replied, "Then I guess I must have just imagined it." Thus, the subjective reality of the experience was so great that even in the waking state he expected physical manifestations of it.

One of our subjects (K) was told that, at the starting signal, she would discuss some problem or decision with some friends, and would come to a definite conclusion concerning it. The topic discussed was to be some actual question with which she was faced, but she was assured that the experimenter would not ask her what it was, and that he did not wish to know. She reported that she had discussed a problem for a half hour or so with several friends, and had reached a decision.

Some months later, she told the experimenter that the problem she had discussed concerned the completion of a house that she and her brother had started for her mother. Her brother had been unable to meet his part of the financial obligations, and she had been faced with the decision as to whether to arrange a loan and complete the house, or to sell her interest in it. She reported that, "My friends advised me to complete it, and I wonder if you will lend me the money to go down to —— in order to make arrangements with the finance company."

The experimenter, on hearing this, explained to her that the only "advice" she could possibly receive from her hallucinated friends originated in her own mind, and he cautioned her against acting on such advice in the future. Her reply was, "Well, they seemed to know what they were talking about, and the advice seemed to be very good." The loan for bus fare was gladly made, and the house was financed and completed, and, fortunately, everything turned out most satisfactorily. That the hallucinated experience must have been very real, to the subject, goes without saying.

Further evidence along these lines is seen in the following case. The experimenter told a subject (J) that one of the things that intrigued him (the experimenter) most was the question as to what a hallucination, as such, is actually made of (meaning the "stuff" of which it is composed). "For instance," he said, "what was that swimming pool that you were diving into actually made of?" The subject's reply was, "It was made just like any other pool, Doc." This answer stresses the pool's realness, to the subject, who inadvertently had completely missed the intended meaning of the question.

In another instance (subject K) the experimenter, anxious to determine whether it required effort on her part to produce the contents of her hallucinated world, or whether they appeared spontaneously, said, "I want to know whether it is an effort for you to have these experiences." The reply was, "Sometimes it is." Asked to elaborate on her answer, she said, "Well, for instance, when you had me see a basketball game the other day, I wasn't ready when my boy friend called for me, and I had to hurry with my bath and my nails so as not to keep him waiting too long." Here again, she misconstrued the question in a way that attests the realness, to her, of the experience.

On the other hand, to the incompletely trained subject, the feeling of reality tone is not necessarily present. Most interesting is the following report from subject N who, incidentally, had an analytical mind, and could express herself with great clarity.

She had been doing work on motor learning which involved the actual waking playing of a piano piece after hallucinated practice, in the trance state, under time distortion.

E. As you sat down at the piano to play, after trance practice, did you have a feeling that you could do it, or not?
S. It was different in the trance.
E. In what way?
S. There were more distractions when I was awake, because I was worried whether I could do it or not, and that didn't affect me in the trance. In the trance, I could hear the music, and my hands would play. Even if they played the wrong notes, I didn't have the "jar" of hearing the wrong notes. I could only tell they were wrong by the feel. The sound—I kept hearing it over and over and it never stopped. And all the time I was hearing I would fumble around, sort of, until I could coordinate the feel of the keys and the sound. And that's the difference between the. . . It's like two separate processes in the trance—the hearing, and the feeling, so that when I sit down to the piano *really*, I still have the feel, but the sound in my

mind is overshadowed by the sound that comes out of the piano. In the trance, I feel that I have some control over the feel and the sound, but I have no control over the real piano (when awake). I feel that I'm really the agent. It's me imagining the sounds, and it's me feeling for the keys. So the music that results is more like I was the instrument, and the whole thing is just a matter of coordination of my own faculties.

E. Did you have the feeling that you had actually been playing?

S. Yes—after I woke up and before I sat down at the piano, I had the feeling that I had been playing. But these keys (of the real piano) were harder and colder, and they didn't even feel quite the same size. On waking, I realized that I had been in a trance and had remembered something I hadn't thought of for 5 or 6 years. In the trance, I had none of that in my mind at all.

This amazing piece of introspection shows that this partly-trained subject had not yet achieved complete "objectivity" in relation to her hallucinatory productions. Indeed, subjects truly are the "agent" of their experiences in the hallucinatory world, but they seldom realize it.

We have the same subject to thank for the following.

E. Please compare the hallucinated trip you just took with a real trip.

S. In the real trip I was awfully excited, anticipating the unknown. In the trance, I'm excited because I know how much fun we had. In the real thing, I would wonder what we were going to do. That time, in the trance, was spent contemplating what I knew would happen.

We must not generalize from these individual reports, but rather view them as expressions of the personality make-up of the person giving them. Other subjects, for instance, have produced movie "shorts" that were highly entertaining and that they had never seen before. Likewise, they have made up stories, in distorted time, to tell to hallucinated children.

CONTINUITY

Action was continuous in all but a very few hypnotically suggested experiences. This was ascertained by frequent questioning. In fact, the subject himself would usually volunteer information concerning an omission or a skip. When these occurred, there was generally a shifting of scene without apparent transit from one location to the other. Another form would be a "floating" from one place to another instead of walking. One subject did this when she became bored.

In several instances, a shift of scene apparently represented an amnesia, for on being asked to relive the action, the subject reported the missing experience.

The hearing of rather long pieces of music, without omission, by musicians is most suggestive of true continuity. One of our subjects was a skilled professional violinist, and another an accomplished amateur. They frequently reported that there were no omissions in the familiar pieces they heard or played in trance. Other subjects gave similar testimony concerning familiar popular music.

Another point that bespeaks continuity is that injected sound signals invariably arrived during hallucinatory action. In other words, this type of exploration revealed no action-free intervals.

The counting experiments also support the view that continuity is present.

TIME SENSE

In well-trained, "good" subjects, the outstanding facts about their time sense, as revealed by their reports, are the following:

1. The hallucinated activity appears, to the subject, to proceed at a normal or customary rate. It is continuous, without "gaps", and seems "very real".

2. Where a completed activity is experienced, without a suggested personal time (S.P.T.), the seeming duration (S.D.) is appropriate to the amount of activity.

3. Where a suggested personal time is used with a continuous activity, the seeming duration of the activity, or of the interval between the starting and termination signals, will be the same as the suggested personal time.

4. The seeming duration of the interval between metronome strokes can be prolonged, to a predetermined degree, by suggestion.

5. Within limits, completed activities will be finished within the allotted time.

Of considerable interest is the fact that occasionally a subject's hallucinated activity will involve "waiting". Thus, one subject, while at an amusement park, reported that, "At the roller coaster, there was a long line of people, and we had to wait." Even more remarkable was the report of another subject to the effect that on several occasions, while engaged in an activity during distorted time, she found herself thinking how tired the experimenter must get waiting so long for her to finish.

For successful "utilization" of experiential time by increased mental activity it is probably mandatory that the subject be totally unaware of his surroundings and of world time. With some subjects this is difficult at first; with others it is easy. Three of our subjects were apparently helped by a brief talk on the relation between subjective and physical time, the dream being cited as the most familiar example of the variability of the former. The transition period which preceded the full acceptance of "special time" in these subjects was most interesting, as the following accounts will show.

The efforts of these subjects to get away from world time are worthy of note. One of them (F), who said she seemed always to be aware of world time, would hallucinate a weird cellophane covering for herself, into which to "escape". With this pulled down over her, she was able to hear several minutes of music, in normal tempo, during but a few seconds of world time. Her difficulties disappeared one day, and with them the necessity for these odd creations, while she was counting silently the strokes of an hallucinated metronome. She counted 27 metronome strokes in 55 seconds and as she did so, found herself watching a "sky-writing" pilot in the air. She was much impressed with what she saw. "Here I am counting by myself in one kind of time and watching an airplane do fancy loops, and it seemed to me that he had so much time to kill between strokes. He had time to do all kinds of fancy loops and things, and it didn't seem strange at all. If he had been writing a word, which he wasn't, there were enough loops to take care of a six- or seven-letter word." Later she said, "I think the thing that convinced me most (of the reality of another sort of time) was seeing the airplane, and noting how easily, effortlessly, or unhurriedly it was looping in between strokes. He seemed to have so much time to kill. Now I really realize that the thing to do is to relax and accept the fact that there is more than one kind of time."

Another remark that is worthy of record was made by a subject (E) who, while in the trance state, refused to demonstrate the rate at which she picked flowers. When asked why she couldn't do so, she said, "I'll try, but I tell you I picked 145 in 10 minutes and I can't repeat it now because I don't have a time limit right now—neither a time limit nor a limit on the flowers I might pick. It doesn't coincide. But there I'm in a certain frame of mind—and it can't be repeated here. I can't do it incomplete—in a fragment. It's impossible. I can do it again too!"

Then, after waking, she said, "Well, I consider this a unique experience with a certain time limit and a certain amount of work to be accomplished. If the time limit or the amount of work or both are eliminated, it is not the same experience any more, so I can't show you in a fragment how it went, or how it was."

Some weeks later she was crystal-gazing in a trance and was asked to see herself picking the same flowers, and to count them aloud as she did so. Under these circumstances she readily complied. The demonstrated rate was 42 per minute.

Another subject (C), in the transition period, once tried to escape world time by "going off from the main shaft of a mine". His difficulties were further revealed in the following remarks:

S. Here's a funny thing now. I was conscious that the physical time was perhaps 11 seconds, but the hallucinated time seemed to be about two minutes. And I was able to move these marbles, one at a time, without taking a handful or anything like that and without hurrying.

E. Were you aware then of two time factors?

S. Yes—I was aware of the consciousness of physical time and also of hallucinated time.

E. Would it be fair to say that you weren't completely lost in the hallucinated experience?

S. No—I was engrossed in the hallucinated experience but yet some other factor seemed to indicate that it was merely 10 or 11 seconds.

E. Were you aware of that while you were counting marbles?

S. No—but when I said (while reporting) "two minutes", the other factor came into play and gave a quiver—a physical shock— to my body, and then the idea of 11 or 10 seconds came.

In some of the tests the subjects spontaneously hallucinated a watch or a clock. In others, these instruments were suggested to them. Usually, but not always, the time indicated by the hallucinated timepieces was appropriate to the subjects' experience.

The following is subject J's answer to a request that he tell how he learned to distort time, during his training:

"At the start, forget everything else. Just do what he (the experimenter) told you to do. Concentrate strictly on what you're going to do.

You start on the task assigned and only that. Don't think about the time. Before you know it, the task is over with, and it seems like a long period of time, and you try to recall where you were—'Where have I been? Where am I?' As soon as your mind gets on the task, and you're doing it, it feels very real. Then you wonder why you've stopped, and you want to go back and retrace what you've done. And it seems like a long time, a very long period of time—maybe 15 or 30 minutes. Like you're dreaming and wake up, you feel you've been wherever your dream is, and then realize you've been in bed. Your mind may run over a lot of things in addition to the task. Sometimes I don't write as much as you say I should. I say, 'I can do it well now.' So I stop. Then I might just wait, or I might do many things—you don't know what. It may seem a month—maybe a month. Lots of thoughts and scenes go through. They may jump from one thing to another, like in a dream. They go faster. But the task itself went at regular or usual speed."

It should be noted that the above account contains evidence that, during training, the subject was aware of both "special time" and world time, as was the case with several of the others.

A very thoughtful and intelligent subject (N) made the following remarks about her experiences with time distortion:

"I can see the beginning and the end of everything I do in a trance. Like a dream, it's a round thing—it's not a progression. In music you have to begin at the beginning and play it through to the end, but in a painting you can see it all at once. In the shorthand things (she was working on the hallucinated writing of shorthand symbols) I'm not as sure of the end."

She went on to say, "That doesn't make sense. I was going to say that they were the same, but they weren't. After the signal, I have the feeling of the whole experience, and then I can go from the general to the particular. In that way I don't skip. Before I had had practice, little tiny things would hold me up, and I'd have to exert effort to get by them."

The subject was, at this period in her training, working with an allotted time of 10 seconds. She was able, with familiar activities such as riding horseback, or dining in a restaurant, to have 20 minutes of continuous experience under these circumstances. But when it came to the hallucinated writing of a shorthand symbol many times, she could not complete the task.

While we were discussing this difficulty, she said, "I might try seeing the beginning and the end, as I do with, say, the other sort of activities." We decided to try this method, and assigned her the task of seeing a whole page of a given symbol, and then to trace them. This met with partial success, as will be seen in her report:

S. I saw the page—the symbol was "these". So I went back and traced it over.

E. How many were there?

S. About a hundred.

E. Could you feel your hand writing it?

S. Yes.

E. How long did it seem to take you?

S. I don't know. Not very long.

E. Did you hurry?

S. Yes.

E. Why?

S. I couldn't pin them down. They weren't very clear, and I wanted to get them written so they wouldn't fade out.

By no means do all subjects have such difficulties as cited in this section. It is indeed fortunate that some of them do, however, because such reports give us an insight into the nature of hallucinatory productions in distorted time that could be obtained in no other way. One idea that suggests itself is that, somewhere in the unconscious, patterns are elaborated as wholes from elements or units assembled from past experience, and that, at the level of experience, these patterns are "lived through" at a normal or customary rate as far as the subject is concerned, yet with extreme rapidity relative to world time.

HALLUCINATIONS AND DREAMS

We do not consider these hypnotically induced experiences to be identical with dreams, and have never used the word "dream" in a suggestion unless we wish to produce such an entity. That our subjects were, in most cases, aware of a difference is evidenced by the fact that they occasionally, while resting, would say, "I went to sleep and had a dream." However, these dreams had no connection with the experimental work. Between assignments it was customary to give the suggestion, "Now let your mind wander whither it will—to pleasant scenes," in response to which they usually engaged in desultory hallucinated activity, which they did not consider the same as dreaming.

Five of our subjects were asked to compare these two types of activity, and all felt that there were differences. Their remarks follow.

Concerning hallucinated activities in hypnosis:

Hallucinations are,

"... better organized."

"... more real than dreams."

"... directed dreams."

"... very true to life, and the experiences carry on as if they were really happening."

"You are conscious of what you are doing and can control the situation better."

"They make sense whereas dreams are often silly and impossible."

Concerning dreams:

Dreams are,

"... less meaningful."

"... often far-fetched."

"They contain nonsense and extraneous things."

"They show less continuity."

"They contain something impossible or unreal."

"In dreams the mind jumps from one subject to another and it is as if the dreamer were looking on instead of participating in it."

"Most dreams are next to impossible."

AWARENESS OF SURROUNDINGS

The subjects with the best performance all reported that while engaged in an assignment they were completely unaware of their surroundings. The ones who were unable to lose touch completely with the physical world had difficulties with time distortion.

ALLOTTED TIME

The relation of the allotted time to the hallucinated experience is a most interesting one.

It has already been pointed out that, during training, if we repeat a given assignment, using a shorter and shorter allotted time with each repetition, the subject will fit the experience into the shortened allotted time without its being changed in any way. This is true whether the task be a completed one, or a continuous one with a suggested personal time. Thus, a subject may hallucinate the writing of a certain word 30 times in an allotted time of 10 seconds at the first assignment, and, at the second, have the same experience, proceeding at the same rate as far as he is concerned, in an allotted time of three seconds.

Again, we may assign as a task the taking of a 20-minute walk, and have the subject tell us when he has finished. Thus, no allotted time is used. The subject, after, say, 218 seconds, tells us that he has finished the walk. Next, let us assign the identical task, but this time we tell the subject that we shall notify him to stop when the 20 minutes are up. Thus we use an allotted time here, and shall assume that it is 10 seconds. A good subject will have completed the assignment at the termination signal, without hurrying, and it will be identical to the previous experience. There will be no difference, in the hallucinated activity as such, between the early portion of the walk and the later portion.

We have no explanation for this ability of the subject to have, within limits, identical experiences, or similar "amounts" of experience, in different world time intervals. There is no evidence that these hallucinated experiences *ordinarily* take place instantaneously relative to world time. On the contrary, the injecting of sound signals, some of the counting experiments, and the inability of subjects to complete an activity if the allotted time is too short, all indicate that the activities are extended in world time. However, in some cases it would seem that, at the termination signal, a previously unfinished task may be completed almost instantaneously relative to world time, and yet in regular tempo as far as the subject himself is concerned. And the well-trained subject will operate with amazingly brief allotted time intervals, as in the case of subject K, who watched an entire basketball game in the interval between two hand-claps placed as close together as the experimenter could place them.

TABLE 7

Controls

SUBJECT	MAXIMUM ERROR (%)
Estimation of short intervals (10–30 seconds)	
C	120
D	85
E	100
F	150
G	100
H	66
Estimation of long intervals (15 minutes to several hours)	
C	80
D	30
E	—
F	25
G	25
H	25

MISCELLANEOUS

The subjects all said that the hallucinated activity never started before the starting signal, and that it invariably ended abruptly at the termination signal.

As an example of the sudden cessation of action, one subject told how the signal came as he was reaching for something, and his hand was in mid-air as the hallucination disappeared.

Aside from their intrinsic significance, these findings speak against retrospective falsification.

CONTROLS

Table 7 shows the ability of a group of our subjects to estimate both short and long world-time intervals while engaged in various activities, in the waking state.

With the short intervals, which varied from 10 to 30 seconds, the activities were counting small objects, sorting cards, talking, and reading. The instructions, incidentally, were patterned after those used under hypnosis in assigning activities. With the longer intervals, ranging from 15 minutes to several hours, ordinary daily occupations were engaged in.

It is quite obvious from the results in table 7 that the estimated times are in far closer agreement with the actual world-time intervals than under the type of time distortion studied in this report.

CHAPTER 15

Association

The following experiments were performed in order to determine whether the process of association could be facilitated by the use of time distortion in hypnosis.

GROUP 1

Activity instructions: "On hearing a word, which I shall say, you will have an experience."

Allotted time: 10 seconds. The word itself constituted the starting signal.

Suggested personal time: none.

Reporting: No spoken report was asked for. On waking, the subject was given a list of the words and described her experiences in writing. Tasks were assigned in groups of ten daily. In the following reports, the word follows the numeral designating the task. We present a fairly large number of these because they convey such a clear impression of the sort of hallucinatory experience with which we are dealing.

1. JAVA—I saw a picture of a group of islands, one of which was Sumatra, and kept trying to see if *Java* was there but couldn't find it or, that is, it wouldn't stay put. Once I would seem to locate it some place and look away; and when I looked back it would seem to have disappeared.

2. TRIBE—We were dancing the squaw dance but I couldn't learn how.

3. FLOCK—I saw a snapshot of myself at age five standing very dressed up at the edge of a huge *flock* of chickens. (The snapshot is real, and I haven't seen it for about 20 years, as all my pictures were lost when we moved.)

4. LITHUANIAN—We were at a party and some men eating little dried fish kept calling each other "Brother *Lithuanian*". They kept laughing and I tried to find out what the joke was and they would offer me some of the fish.

5. HALF—My mother was trying to get admitted to an Indian hospital for treatment and the admitting nurse asked for proof that she was

83

¼ Indian. My mother said she was ½. "One-*half* is not one-fourth," said the nurse, and my mother just looked at me helplessly but I couldn't think of any good argument.

6. FIFTH—I saw a colonial-type building with great white pillars. I was looking at the top to see what kind of architecture they were. The *fifth* one seemed to be different, but I was unable to analyze the difference, though I was sure there was some if I'd keep looking.

7. THREE—I saw a station-wagon with "*Three* Sisters Ranch" lettered on the side and wondered if it were mine, but I decided not to get in it.

8. ENOUGH—My sister and I were acting silly and giggling. My mother kept saying "That's enough. That's enough." Pretty soon she spanked us and when we cried, said, "That's *enough* crying," and spanked us some more. I went out under the persimmon tree and hated her.

9. ALL—I was doing beadwork on a buckskin purse. I wanted to make my own design and choose my own colors, but the lady who was teaching me made the choice for me. Although the beads were *all* sizes and I had to keep sorting them to make them fit the design, it turned out very well and I was most pleased.

10. FEW—I heard the phrase "*few* succeed" running over and over in my mind and tried to connect it with something. Finally I decided it has something to do with crossing an imaginary line, not physical, but color, racial or social.

11. THE—I was in the living room of my home and my mother was teaching me to read. It was very repetitious material—"Hop, hop went the little bird. *The* little bird hopped." She had me pronounce "the" with a long e, not "thuh".

12. THIS—(This, that.) These words came to me together on the suggestion of "this", and I was in a car riding from Gallup to Albuquerque with a man who was a mediator from the Labor Department. He gave me a long lecture on the inefficiency of most people's vocabulary, how important it was to know the proper words to fit the proper places, and how meaningless to fill your talk with "and thus and so", "and *this* and *that*", and "Whatchamacallit".

13. SUCH—I was baking a pie by a new recipe and the crust was all crumbly and wouldn't stay together, though I kept adding water.

14. AN—I was about eight, and had just read from a large book a silly phrase which I kept repeating, enjoying its silliness and continuity, "*An* Illinoisy noisy noise annoys a noisy oyster." I had the measles and wasn't supposed to be reading.

15. SOME—I was on a bus with the wind blowing in the open window. The people sitting behind me were talking, the one not loud enough to distinguish her voice but the other would say now and again in a loud,

I-told-you-so tone, "Well, *some* do, and *some* don't." First I kept trying to study, but finally gave up and tried to hear, to no avail.

16. I—I saw *myself* as a little girl reciting the pledge of allegiance to the flag to my father. The first time I was just memorizing it. The next time was several years later and I had grown quite a bit.

17. THOU—An old farmer was kneeling down in the mud getting ready to pray when a preacher came around the side of the house and said, "You don't need to pray there, so long as you're willing to."

18. HE—A little girl was walking by, pulling petals off daisies, saying, "He loves me, he loves me not." Each time she would end with "He loves me not" and start on a new one. I gave her some more, and as she walked away, she seemed to be having better luck, ending with the positive statement louder and with finality.

19. SHE—My cousin Ethel was visiting us when I was seven years old. Every place we went people would exclaim, "Isn't *she* beautiful?" I thought so, too, and she became my idol right then, but she walked away and never came back.

20. WE—I was studying, trying to define the feeling of "in-group" to myself so I could state it in words. I thought, "It's a feeling of 'we-ness', but will anyone understand what I mean by that? Then I thought, it's the difference between thinking of myself separately rather than "Here *we* are together."

21. YOU—A barmaid was pointing to a handwritten sign on a door, "Please Close Door" and underneath, "This Means U." She said, "You don't know how much effect that last phrase has. We had that sign 'Please Close Door' up for months and the door was never closed. As soon as I added 'This Means U', everyone started closing it."

22. THEE—I had just received a telephone call from Dick and was dressing to go out, puzzling over why I had never noticed before that he used "thee" in direct address, or if he really didn't but I had just heard him wrong that time. I listened particularly for it later, but could not detect it.

23. MY—I saw *my*self age fourteen hugging a little dog. I was living with friends, and the little dog was the first thing that I felt had ever belonged to me to not have to share with sisters, and I was fiercely possessive about him.

24. ME—There were try-outs for a school play being given and I wanted one part desperately and had studied the part quite carefully. However, when it came my turn, the teacher wouldn't let me say my lines but told *me* to sing instead. I tried, but no one could hear me and I went on feeling very small and inadequate.

25. THY—I was very small, about three, and my mother was sitting

in a big high-backed rocker teaching me to read from a big Bible. When I did well, she would give me round colored candies which I'd put in a small jar and save.

26. His—My father had just returned from a trip and we were anxiously waiting for him to open *his* grip to see what he had brought. When he opened it, it smelled so good of shaving creams, etc. Then he gave us the candy he'd brought, and let me look at the gun he always carried which had a buffalo-head carved ivory handle.

27. Their—While I was riding on a train, an Indian couple got on. They were so pleased with themselves I started watching them now and again, glancing up from my book. It was getting close to my stop, so I started eyeing my luggage to know where it all was when I saw there was another black bag just like mine. I was wondering which was *their* bag when the man asked the woman in a distinct voice with an Indian accent, "Whirs the sootcase," and she answered by pointing with her lips and saying, "It's over there."

28. Herself—"D", a neighbor in Yankton, was calling to her little girl, "Don't run. You'll hurt yourself." I felt sorry for the little girl, for I thought "She's not afraid she'll hurt *herself*, she's just afraid she'll get her white shoes dirty."

29. This—I was working in my flower garden, sort of sitting on my haunches and reaching close to the house to pull weeds when I felt something cool and smooth with my hand. I drew it out and it was a pretty apple-green snake. I put it down and it slowly crawled away.

30. Which—I was telling a little girl that I thought I would just have a sandwich for dinner. She inquired, "What's a sand*witch*?" "Don't be silly, Patty, you know what a sandwich is. You have them for lunch every day," I said. "But I was thinking of a 'witch,' you know," she said, and smiled.

31. That—I was walking by Aunt Rosie's chicken yard and there by the side of it was a cow seemingly wearing a lady's straw hat. When she chewed, the cherries on it would bounce. I looked back as I went on, and the cow was still there wearing the hat.

32. Those—I had an apartment in a private home and just as I was getting ready to go out, Mrs. D. called accusingly, "You didn't water the lawn today," and while I was trying to decide whether to go back and do it or go on and catch my bus, sprinklers sprang up all over the lawn and got me all wet, so I just walked on toward the bus.

33. Kill—I was on my grandmother's farm when the hired men were going over to the pigpen early in the morning. I ran after them and they chased a little pig and cut its throat, and it ran around dizzily squealing

and spurting blood. I felt kind of sorry for it, but they said it ate smaller little pigs, so then I was glad.

34. SLEEP—I was in a hospital in a room with blue walls; I kept hearing a sweeping sound, and a nurse was trying to wake me to wash, but I didn't want to wake up and kept trying to stay *asleep*.

35. LIFT—I was watching the burning of Zozobra, and as he gave his last cry and collapsed, I felt a certain freedom as though a weight had been *lifted* from my mind.

36. LEAVE—I was counting, counting and re-counting to see if I had enough *leave* to cover the vacation I wanted to take. When I found I probably hadn't, I decided to request LWOP and quit worrying about it.

37. SLEEPING—I seemed to be *sleeping* in a great pine forest on a bed of pine needles. The scent of pine was heavy and the wind sighed through the trees just as I'd always heard. I must have been only half-asleep, because I was conscious of these things and of enjoying them and thinking, "I must find out where I am so that I can come back."

38. COME—I am about four or five years old, am at my grandmother's funeral, and people are singing, "Come, come, come. . . " I thought it was a very pretty song and wished they would sing it at our church.

39. FOUND—My mother had sent me to the garden to pick potato bugs, and I was hating every minute of it. Suddenly I looked down and saw I had *found* a ruby ring I had lost years ago. I was most excited, and put it on immediately to see if it still fit, which it did, and was as good as new.

40. EAT—I was about 12, was visiting a family friend and sitting out back of her house *eating* a sandwich she had made for me. I was very hungry, and was wondering whether I might ask for another as I had never had one at home that tasted so good. Then my mother came outside and was ready to go home.

41. FLOW—It was late November and I was sitting on a beach in San Francisco alone watching the ebb and *flow* of the water and feeling a little cold.

42. BLOW—I was sitting in the living room in a friend's house and her husband was teaching me to *blow* smoke-rings. Suddenly I felt very ill and was embarrassed about it, so I said I had to see Agnes about something and rushed upstairs and lay on the bed for quite a while.

43. GRAZE—I was sitting in a car near Ft. Defiance idly watching some sheep *grazing* and thinking how dirty sheep were, and wishing I dared ask the Navajo to show me how they fixed their hair.

These experiences were all continuous and very "real". Their seeming duration was from 5 minutes to several hours.

Free association was tested in the following tasks:

Waking: The subject was told that a word would be said to her and that this would bring to mind another word, and then another, and so on. In 30 seconds she wrote the following in response to the word "barrel": stave, rainwater, mosquitoes, fever, temperature, thermometer, get well.

Trance state: Activity instructions: "I shall say a word to you. This word will bring to mind another word, and then another, and so on. This will go on for at least 10 minutes. The word is baby."

Allotted time: 10 seconds.

Suggested personal time: at least 10 minutes.

Report: No spoken report was asked for. On waking, she wrote the following: baby, boy, shoes, run, fall down, hill, Jack and Jill, hurry, library, bookshelves, 3 cents, gum, steal, neighbor, road, cull, telephone, Cecil, dress, flowers, dance, James, wrestle, grit teeth, get, look fierce, win, shooting, sun, doctor, trial, devil.

Asked to describe the process, she said, "They were scenes. I would see something like a little boy, and the word would come. Then I'd see white shoes on him, and the word 'shoes' would come. Then I'd see him running, and the word 'run' would come."

On another occasion the subject reported 40 or 50 associations. The allotted time was 10 seconds, suggested personal time 10 minutes, and seeming duration 5 minutes. She was not asked to write them out, but the following report was obtained:

E. Did you think of things?
S. Yes.
E. How long did it seem?
S. I don't know, about five minutes.
E. Did you have many associated thoughts?
S. Yes. It went more jagged. The other was all orderly and progressive. This started as an orderly progression. Then it jumped around. There was a kind of progression, but not much.
E. In what form did these associations come to you?
S. Well, it seemed like it was what you call experiences, because it seemed like I was there.
E. Did you recognize any actual experiences you'd had before?
S. Yes.
E. Were you the same age all through?
S. No.

E. Was there any sexual material involved?

S. No.

E. Can you give me the roughest sort of an estimate as to how many experiences there were?

S. Oh, 40 or 50.

E. Now, as you think of this task, do any questions arise in your mind?

S. No.

E. Was there an emotional content to any of these experiences?

S. Mostly a kind of pleasant feeling, but not—not any deep emotion one way or another.

E. Were any of the experiences such as would be accompanied by pronounced emotion in the waking state if you actually had them?

S. No, I don't think so, although in the beginning one was connected with a funeral. I was young. I might have been emotional, but for children I guess those things are more of a social affair.

E. What was the youngest age at which you found yourself?

S. I was a child in one of the scenes but I was not aware of my age. That scene went on for quite a while. Then, in the next, it skipped until I was about 22, and that didn't last very long.

DISCUSSION BY MILTON H. ERICKSON

In first reading the above accounts, the question arises at once concerning the validity of the reported associations. Were they actually the result of the experiment and did they occur in distorted time? Or do they represent a combination of such associations with an admixture of unwitting waking associations occasioned by the very process of reporting in the waking state? Should the latter be the case, while it would not invalidate the associations themselves as meaningful to the subject, it would pose the experimental problem of differentiating associations developed in time distortion from those arising from waking activity.

However, careful reading of the accounts discloses a significant and markedly consistent pattern. This is that, in practically every account, the experience lies not in the narrative words used in reporting but in the experiential and time duration implications of the account. Personal problems involving time and characterized by doubt, uncertainty, repetitious effort, frustration, waiting, tension, decisions, ambivalences, etc. mark the majority of the reports. Furthermore, the duration of the time implied is beyond that needed for the narrative significance.

For example, in Task 5, the first two sentences constitute a simple narration. The last sentence is a statement of an experiential problem embracing doubt, uncertainty, frustration and requiring time and repeated effort. In Task 13, the narrative concerned baking a pie by a new recipe with the crust "all crumbly". The experiential and time duration aspects are expressed by the implications of the words "and it wouldn't stay together though I kept adding water to it." And the account of Task 32, in addition to illustrating similar significances, suggests strongly the additional item of a dream experience.

The report of the experiment on free association is similarly significant. The results secured by the waking control activity were those ordinarily elicited. The trance activity in time distortion was of another character entirely, both in kind and extent, although the actual temporal duration was only a third as long. It was not only much more extensive but it was very greatly elaborated. Instead of free association by words, whole scenes were utilized from which a single word was abstracted to meet the demand of the experimental situation. In addition, a sense of participation in the scenes, either as a spectator or as an actor, was reported, with the subject experiencing the self at a wide range of age levels.

While these experiments are not sufficiently extensive to warrant definitive conclusions, the significances of the results obtained are highly indicative that time distortion can be utilized to facilitate the association of ideas. Out of such association can come the recovery of forgotten and repressed memories.

CHAPTER 16

Thought

All our subjects felt that the thought processes they employed in their hallucinations were comparable to those of the waking state. In fact, some of them felt that they were possibly of a superior type, there being an increased ability to consider situations as a whole. One said, "Considerations are weighed out mentally instead of verbally." We were, unfortunately, unable to give this matter the attention it deserved.

We feel that this is true thought. If such indeed be the case, then it is obvious that this all-important mental activity, at least a form of it, can take place at very rapid rates, while appearing to proceed normally. It is obvious also that such thought can deal only with concepts available through memory. Yet it is possible that the increased accessibility of material from the unconscious might be advantageous under certain circumstances.

Three sorts of tasks were assigned in investigating the ability of subjects to employ thought during time distortion in hypnosis.

1. THE SOLVING OF HYPOTHETICAL PROBLEMS NOT INVOLVING MATHEMATICS, AND IDEATION CONCERNING SPECIFIC QUESTIONS

In these tasks, the subject was presented with a problem to consider, and given both an allotted time (10 seconds) and a suggested personal time (10 minutes) for its completion. The following example will illustrate the technique:

"I'm going to give you a problem to solve in ten minutes. After I tell you the problem you will receive a signal, at which you will start working on it. At the end of ten minutes I shall give you the signal to stop. You will have plenty of time.

"Now here is the problem. A young girl is in love with a young man who wants to marry her. However, the girl has an invalid mother who is dependent upon her, and to whom she feels obligated. She hesitates to marry because she does not wish to burden her fiance with her mother, and yet she is very anxious to get married and does not wish to sacrifice her entire life to her mother. These young people want your advice.

"When I give you the signal you're going to think this situation over from all points of view and afterwards tell me what conclusion you came to.

"Here comes the signal—Start."

Ten seconds, world time, later she was told, "Time is up. Now tell me about the problem."

The subject reported that she saw and talked to a young man and a girl about this, their problem. She discussed the matter at length with them, asking the girl various questions and receiving answers. She suggested that the girl work after marriage in order to support her mother, who, she felt, should not live with the young people but rather with some friend her own age. She did not think that the girl should give up her life to her mother, but on the other hand, she shouldn't shirk her responsi-bility. She should marry by all means. She talked mostly to the girl. "The boy didn't have much to say."

Her account of this experience was amazing in the fullness of detail and the amount of reflection that it apparently indicated. This was especially surprising in view of the fact that in waking life the subject is not prone to speculate on matters. When told that she had thought the problem through, not in ten minutes but rather in ten seconds, she was astounded.

Numerous other problems were presented from time to time, among them the following:

Should a young girl, daughter of well-to-do parents, seek a job?

What are the relative merits of government and private industry employment?

Are you in favor of compulsory military training?

What do you think about segregation of the Negro in the South?

In every case the reports gave evidence of careful and thorough consideration, and the estimated personal time interval was always the same as the suggested one. She didn't have to hurry. She always "saw" something—that is, she saw and talked to the young couple; she saw the girl who was discussing the job; she saw a government office building and a factory; in considering the Negro problem she was watching a group of poor and shabby Negroes in a small southern town. A fish-bowl with names in it appeared while she was considering compulsory military training.

The last test done was given a suggested personal time of 10 minutes, but an allotted time of only three seconds. The subject reported that she seemed to be working on it for ten minutes, and gave a very complete account of her "thoughts".

Counseling tasks, assigned to psychology students, would also fall in this group.

2. THE PREPARATION OF BRIEF LECTURES, AND THEIR DELIVERY, OR THE MAKING UP OF STORIES

A sample of the former is the following task assignment: "When I give you the starting signal, by saying 'Now', you will spend 20 minutes preparing an outline for a short talk to a group of senior high school students. The topic will be, 'Psychology as a Career'. Now." Subject I was used for a small group of such experiments, using an allotted time of five seconds. As a control, a similar task was assigned to him in the waking state, with the same allotted time. With the trance tasks, he accepted the S.P.T. in full, and was able to do a good deal of orderly thinking, although this was not fully appropriate to the S.P.T. Asked to comment on his waking performance as compared to the trance activity, he replied, "There's no comparison. I hardly got started (in the waking task)."

Such tasks involve a re-ordering of elements from past experience, and thus constitute, in a sense, creative thought. The same is true of the production of movie "shorts" never before seen, in distorted time. Some of the comedies, or animated cartoons, were quite amusing and were enjoyed by the subjects. The making up of stories involving stipulated characters is another example of this sort of creative activity. With these, a sample suggestion would be, ". . . you're going to make up a story about a horse, an old woman, and a ship." This type of task is, of course, familiar to everyone, for everyone has had a child ask him, "Please tell me a story." The hallucinatory drawing of pictures falls into this category also.

3. THE SOLVING OF MATHEMATICAL PROBLEMS

This is discussed in Chapter 20.

CHAPTER 17

Creative Mental Activity

The following experiment was run in order to investigate the possibility that creative mental activity can be facilitated under conditions of time distortion in hypnosis.

SUBJECT

The subject (M) was a secretary who was also going to college, where she was majoring in psychology. She had long been interested in dress designing and possessed considerable talent in the field.

DESIGNING IN THE WAKING STATE

Her written account of her customary approach to designing a dress follows:

"When I have decided that I want to design a dress, I usually look around at dresses in shop windows and at pictures of dresses in newspapers and magazines, and I may look at material. And I usually over-buy the material because I am not sure yet how I'm going to make it. I take the material and play with it awhile and drape it on me. Then I generally start cutting muslin patterns. When I have a basic pattern that pleases me, I cut out the material and make the dress, deciding on the details as I go along. Sometimes I draw as I go along, but I never draw the whole thing. It's sort of a working tool, not a design to work from. I often work intermittently over a period of several months, sometimes for several hours at a time on from four to ten occasions."

As a control, we twice assigned to her in the waking state the task of designing a dress. In the first case, she left her desk at the end of a half hour and said, "I'm just wasting my time because I can't think of anything about anything. I don't have one single idea." In the second, she likewise produced nothing in the course of a half hour. Her written report on what she did was, "I sat there and thought or, more precisely, tried to think, but the only things I thought of at all were newspaper or magazine pictures of dresses. I can't just sit down and design something, and I never attempt to because I know it is useless."

DESIGNING IN THE TRANCE STATE UNDER CONDITIONS OF TIME DISTORTION

Activity instructions: These were the same in all the tasks, and were as follows: "When I give you the starting signal by saying 'Now', you're going to design a dress. You'll have all the time you need."

Allotted time: This varied from ten seconds to one second.

Suggested personal time: "You'll have all the time you need."

This task was assigned six times. No spoken report was taken in any instance. The subject was waked immediately after the completion of each trance activity and asked to draw a picture of the dress she had designed and to describe it briefly. In task 1, the picture was not requested These reports follow:

Task 1

"I had some beige taffeta shantung but not enough to do what I wanted. I kept thinking and measuring the material, and finally decided I could accomplish what I wanted by making the dress a straight sheath, and using the remaining material cut from the side to make a pleated collar with long ties. The long ties would make it possible to wear it also as a peplum."

Allotted time: Ten seconds.

Seeming duration: One hour.

Task 2

Allotted time: Ten seconds.

Seeming duration: One hour.

Additional report:

    E. Where were you?

    S. I was at home.

    E. How long did you seem to be working at it?

    S. Oh, about an hour. I was sitting at a table, looking out of the window and thinking.

    E. Did you do some drawing?

    S. Yes, after I had thought it all through.

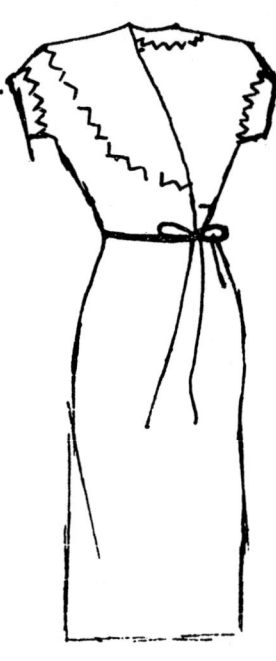

The dress of dark green hopsacking is very slim and plain. The waist had a surplice closing. The collar, of white pique, started very small at the right front of neck, increasing in size as it progressed around neck and down left side of bodice.

Short sleeves have cuffs of white pique.

FIG. 2 (task 2)

Task 3

Allotted time: Five seconds.
Seeming duration: Several hours.
Additional report:

> E. Anything to say about the dress?
> S. No, except that I should like to make it.
> E. Had you ever designed this before?
> S. No.
> E. How long were you working on it?
> S. Several hours, like an afternoon.

Task 4

Allotted time: One second.
Seeming duration: One and a half hours.

Task 5

Allotted time: One second.
Seeming duration. One and a half hours.

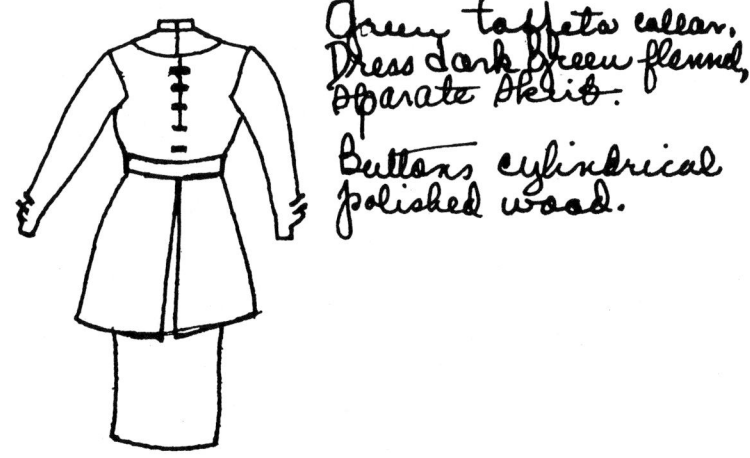

Green taffeta collar. Dress dark green flannel, separate skirt. Buttons cylindrical polished wood.

FIG. 3 (task 3)

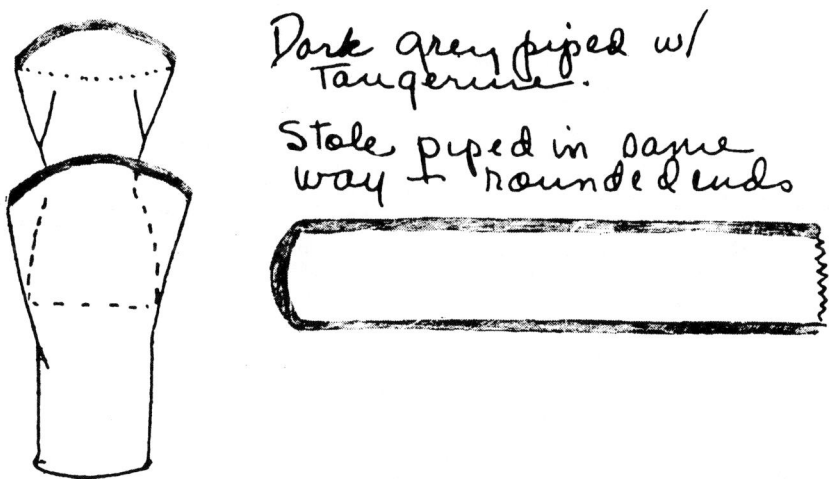

Dark grey piped w/ Tangerine. Stole piped in same way + rounded ends

FIG. 4 (task 4)

Additional report:

E. What do you think of the dress?

S. I like the idea about the belt. The rest I don't think much about one way or the other.

E. Where were you working on it?

S. At home.

E. Did you draw a picture?

S. Yes.

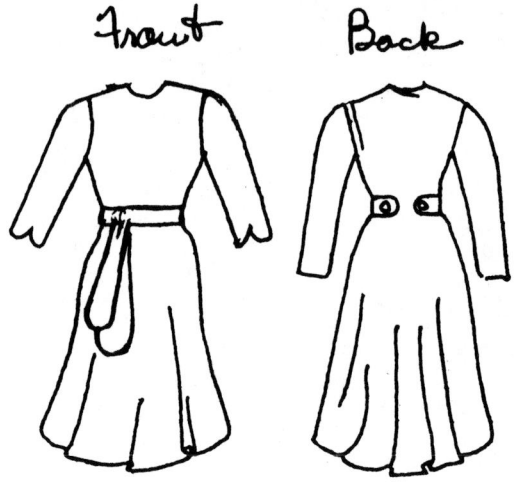

Belt removable - buttons on w/
large buttons in back. Dress
black or navy. One red belt
One of white pique.

FIG. 5 (task 5)

E. Did you hurry?
S. No.

Task 6

Allotted time: Ten seconds.
Seeming duration: One hour.
Additional report:

E. How long did it seem that you were working?
S. Maybe an hour.
E. Did you draw the dress in the trance?
S. No.
E. What did you do?
S. I just thought about it. First I thought about pleats, etc.
E. Did you finish?
S. Yes. I knew what I was going to do.
E. Your surroundings?

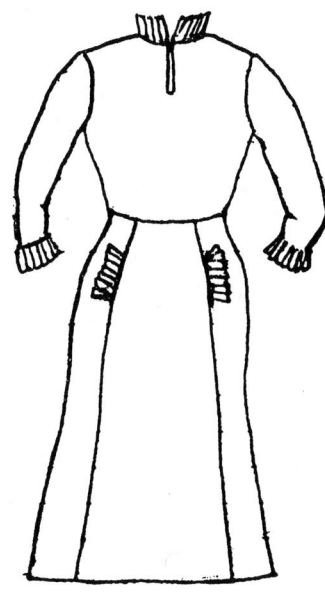

Black lightweight wool.

Sleeves fitted tight at upper forearm

Self-material. pleating on inset pockets around bottom of sleeves and forming stand-up collar.

FIG. 6 (task 6)

S. I was sitting in an easy chair at home. I don't usually use pencil and paper. After I have the dress in mind, I may draw it. Usually I don't draw until after I have made it or started, so I can see how it's going to work.

E. Were you pleased with the dress?

S. Yes.

The subject, on being waked and asked to draw the dresses, went about this with no hesitation whatsoever. It took her about 15 minutes. There is little doubt that she had the idea of the finished dress in mind. In other words, she had already created the design. These designs were all new ones, and she was pleased with the results.

She was asked to compare her experience during one of the half-hour waking tasks with that during trance task 6. Her report follows:

"In comparing the task in the waking state with that carried out in the trance state and recorded in the waking state, I should say that:

"In the waking state I sat there for ages and tried every way I knew how to think of something and could not. While trying to think, I doodled bits of dresses I had seen pictures of, but I never did think of anything that even seemed original in any way.

"In the trance state, my mind seemed clearer and I didn't have to try so hard. I had several ideas which I manipulated until I had what I considered the best combination in my mind. Later I recorded them on paper. The trance activity seemed to last about an hour."

The following is her description of the methods she used in her trance designing:

"In some of them I had material and I sort of worked the design out as I went along. In others, I didn't have the material, and I just thought about the designs, usually starting with the details at the neck and working down. Sometimes I drew them and sometimes I didn't."

DISCUSSION

Of course, no generalizations can be drawn from this one experiment. However, these results suggest that distorted time can be "utilized" for creative mental activity in a field in which the subject is adept.

CHAPTER 18

Motor Learning[1]

As already mentioned, one of our subjects, a professional violinist, became convinced that purely hallucinated practice of previously learned pieces, using her *special trance time*, was helpful to her. In fact, she has since used this method, in a self-induced trance state, for preparing for recitals. Her report of her earlier experiences follows:

"I put myself into a trance and then practiced in several different ways. I might see the music before me and mark the spots that needed extra practice. I would then play the different spots over and over until I got them—which helped my finger memory because I was actually playing in the trance." (This was hallucinated activity only. In other words, she was "actually playing" only in the hallucinated world and not in the physical world.)

"I did 'passage practice'—picking hard passages and playing them in several ways to facilitate speed and accuracy."

"Then I went through the whole composition for continuity. In doing this in 'special time' I seemed to get an immediate grasp of the composition as a whole."

Thus, allegedly, she was able to practice and review long pieces over and over in very brief *world time* periods, and she found that not only did her memory improve strikingly, but also her technical performance. This remarkable result is attested to by her husband, himself a musician. In other words, she felt that purely hallucinated practice of these pieces, in distorted time, improved her subsequent performance.

This naturally led us to further inquiry into this subject, and into the possible use of a similar method for learning *new* motor skills. There are, incidentally, several reports in the literature (13, 16, 19) of the effectiveness of "imaginary practice" in the acquisition of such skills in the wak-

---

[1] Reprinted, with some changes, from "Time Distortion in Hypnosis and Motor Learning", by L. F. Cooper and C. H. Tuthill, in Journal of Psychology, 1952, **34**, 67–76.

ing state. Lovatt (12) has reported the use of hallucinatory practice of motor activities in the trance state. Marked time distortion was present.

It should be emphasized here that, during purely hallucinated motor activity under time distortion in hypnosis, the subjects remain motionless throughout. Despite this, they report that they "really participate in the activity" and, on waking, feel just as if they had done so and had acquired the benefit of any practice that might have been involved.

In one subject, an electromyogram was taken during the purely hallucinated practice of subordinate-hand writing and, though there was no grossly discernible motion, action currents were picked up from single motor units, using unipolar needle electrodes placed in a superficial flexor muscle of the thumb.

We know of two interesting cases where motor activity happened to accompany hallucinatory activity under conditions of time distortion.

One of them has been furnished us by a colleague (18). He hypnotized his son and suggested to him that he would see a movie. This suggestion was carried out by the boy during the course of a few minutes. During the hallucinatory activity the father noticed that the boy's hand moved very rapidly from his right knee toward his mouth and back again. On being waked, the boy reported that he had, indeed, seen a movie. When asked why his hand moved as it did, he replied, "I was eating popcorn." It would seem, then, that the motor activity, which proceeded at a rate of two or three movements per second, represented an attempt on the part of a limited portion of the neuromuscular apparatus to produce motion that was synchronous with the hallucinatory activity which was proceeding in distorted time.

Again, Inglis (10) had a subject who delivered a speech, which he had memorized, at a rate of over 400 words a minute. This was recorded on a record and was unintelligible. Interestingly enough, the speaker thought that he was speaking at a normal rate.

The above considerations led us to hypothesize that possibly there is some central synaptic, and at times even peripheral, electrical activity accompanying the hallucination of motor action during distorted time in hypnosis. It has been impossible, to date, to proceed further with electromyographic studies, but this is certainly indicated, for the amount of electrical activity per second might be found to vary directly with the amount of hallucinated action, per second of *world time*.

SUBJECTS

Subjects I, J, K, L and M were used in this experiment.

The subjects in this study were first trained so that they could finish the hallucination of completed activities involving approximately a half-hour's action in an allotted time of 10 seconds, and could experience a suggested personal time interval of 30 minutes as such, and approach the filling of this interval with an appropriate amount of hallucinated activity within an allotted time of 10 seconds.

They were then trained to hallucinate the writing of a word, with the subordinate hand, at least 10 times, in an allotted time of 10 seconds, doing it carefully and without hurrying.

METHOD

The experiment was planned on the theory that a neuromuscular pattern which had been implanted in the waking state might become more deeply impressed by *trance practice* in distorted time. In choosing an experimental activity, it was necessary to select one that did not depend appreciably, for its execution, upon visual space perception. Among such skills considered were typewriting, stenotyping, adding machine operation, knitting, and subordinate-hand writing. The last one was chosen, and proved to be fairly satisfactory.

At each daily session, the subject first sat at a desk and copied once, in pencil, a sentence containing all the letters of the alphabet, as well as a list of from 10 to 20 individual words. His instructions were as follows:

> Please write the sentence and the words with your left hand (in the case of the left-handed subject, right hand). Since useful writing is a compromise between perfect letter-formation and practical speed you will strive to produce good ordinary writing such as you might use in your daily routine. Please "push yourself" a bit so as to encourage progress.

After this *physical writing* was finished, a moderately deep trance state was induced by suggestions of sleep, the subject being seated in an armchair with his eyes closed.

The following suggestion was then given:

> When I give you the starting signal by saying "Now", you will find yourself sitting at a desk with pencil and paper at hand. You will then pick up the pencil and write the words I give you, with your left hand, at least 30 times. You will write exactly as you did

at my desk a bit ago, and will not hurry, for you will have all the time (*special trance time*) that you need. The word is "horse". "Now."

After an *allotted time* interval of from three to 10 seconds, depending upon the subject, the termination signal "Now, blank", was given. This meant to the subject that he was to discontinue all hallucinated activity and make his mind a blank.

The remaining words were then assigned and practiced in an identical way, and then the sentence was given, to be written out 10 times.

Early in the experiment the subject, after being waked, was asked to write the material again. This was subsequently discontinued, as it constituted an increase in the amount of actual physical writing involved. Still later, only a sentence which contained all the letters of the alphabet was assigned for physical writing. Trance practice then involved the repeated writing of the individual letters as well as the words.

Subjects were tested before the experiment began, on several occasions during the experiment, and again at its conclusion. The number of letters copied during the original test served as a "base-line" for measuring future improvement. The instructions for these tests were as follows:

Your performance is now to be tested. You will copy this material, writing with your left hand, for five minutes. I shall tell you when to begin and when to stop. You will attempt to produce good ordinary handwriting, and within this limitation, will work as rapidly as possible. Here comes the signal—"Now".

With one exception, subjects worked one hour daily, Sundays excluded.

RESULTS

All the subjects reported that task performance seemed to be easier following hallucinated practice.

They invariably reported that their purely hallucinated writing seemed very "real", and that after waking they felt as if they had physically written the words, just as they had during the preceding period of physical writing. The amount of this hallucinated writing done increased as the experiment progressed. For the single words, it was never less than 10 repetitions, and sometimes was well over 30. The more proficient subjects averaged between 20 and 30 repetitions. All felt that they had ac-

TABLE 8

	SUBJECT				
	A	B	C	D	E
Improvement (%)............	87	104	21	87	51
Physical writing (letters)......	4,486	3,159	1,712	1,764	660
Physical writing (minutes)....	140	96	52	98	26
Hallucinated writing (min.)...	47	27	32	102	19

quired the same practice effect that they would expect from an equivalent amount of physical writing.

On several occasions, subjects reported fatigue or discomfort in the hand or wrist during hallucinated writing, and two subjects said that this persisted after waking.

Electromyographic studies in one subject showed action currents to be present in a superficial flexor of the thumb during the hallucinated writing.

Table 8 shows the percentage increase in output as related to physical and hallucinated writing. A wide individual variation is apparent in these results.

CONTROLS

Two groups of controls are available. The first is a group from about 75 amputees who were trained in subordinate-hand writing by a therapist at one of the U. S. Army hospitals. Information concerning these individuals was obtained from the person who trained them, and it is to be emphasized that her estimate of the time required is of the most approximate sort, for the training had been done during and shortly after the recent war, and no stress had been placed upon the time element. The patients were tested for performance, however, on various occasions. From among these, the individual to be considered here was mentally normal, in his "late teens" or in his "twenties", free from severe emotional disturbance relative to his disability, with a normal subordinate extremity, and with a high-school or college education. It is the opinion of the above-mentioned instructor that such an individual could be expected to double his 20-minute output of subordinate-hand writing after 30 hours of practice. This practice was usually divided into daily one-hour periods.

The above group leaves much to be desired as a control, even the number of individuals in the category described being unknown. With due allowance for this fact, however, the opinion expressed would indicate a definite advantage for the learning method described in this paper.

Since a definite amount of *physical writing*, in the waking state, was done by our subjects, it is necessary to try to evaluate its contribution to the improvement shown. In order to do this we assigned to a group of five college students the first 1,648 letters of the material used by our subjects. This was copied in subordinate-hand writing, the instructions being the same as those used in the experiment. The material is fairly comparable in amount to that copied by Subjects C and D at the time that they had improved 21 per cent and 87 per cent respectively. These tasks were assigned over a comparable number of days. Unfortunately it was necessary to employ one of our subjects to assign and supervise these tasks, and thus another variable was introduced.

The improvement shown by these controls was 11, 15, 114, 108, and 84 per cent. Thus, it would seem that the mere copying of the material could be sufficient to account for the improvement shown by our subjects.

DISCUSSION

There is no evidence, in the results of this experiment, that the learning process itself is facilitated by *trance practice* under conditions of time distortion in hypnosis.

The very nature of these studies makes proper control most difficult, because individuals vary widely in their ability to acquire new motor skills, and every bit of *physical writing* employed during an experiment of this design contributes to the learning process. Furthermore, the matter of motivation, both in the waking and the trance states, is a variable of great importance, as well as is the interpretation by the subject of the instructions preceding each test of performance.

Possibly the ideal method of studying this problem would be to take a fairly large group of students at the beginning of a course in typing in a secretarial school, train them as our subjects were trained, and then, each day, give them a short period of *trance practice* on material learned that day. This group could then be compared with the rest of the class. Such an experiment would be most interesting, and not specially difficult. It is conceivable, even, that the practice could be assigned to the entire experimental group at one time at the end of each day.

It is difficult to know, in the present experiment, how to interpret the report on the waking-state training of the group of amputees mentioned above. This report, obviously, indicates a definite advantage in favor of *trance practice* in distorted time.

On the other hand, in our own group of special controls, it is quite clear that no such advantage appears. Possibly, practice effects might be demonstrable in a motor skill where the "neuro-muscular pattern" was a bit more solidly implanted than was the case with these subjects, who physically wrote each word but once. The allied question of review of previously solidly learned material, such as a long-neglected piano piece, should be investigated.

SUMMARY

An attempt was made to determine whether the learning of a new motor skill could be facilitated by purely hallucinated practice under conditions of *time distortion* in hypnosis.

The considerations that led up to this inquiry are mentioned.

Five subjects were used. The design of the experiment was to allow the subjects to write words and sentences, once each, with the subordinate hand, while in the waking state. This was done in order to form a definite neuro-muscular pattern. Then, in the trance state, while the subjects remained motionless, and under conditions of *time distortion*, they hallucinated the repeated writing of the words written while awake.

The subjects felt that this purely hallucinated activity was very real, and that they had obtained practice effects comparable to a similar amount of physical writing. The hallucinated writing seemed to proceed at the same rate as the previous *physical writing*, and the experiential time was appropriate. Increased ease was reported during subsequent waking performance.

Progress in learning was measured in terms of the number of letters written in a waking period of five minutes, using a pre-experimental test as the base. This data is tabulated.

A single electromyographic study of one subject during *trance practice* showed action currents in a superficial flexor of the thumb.

The performance of two inadequate control groups is reported.

The findings are discussed, and suggestions offered for future investigations.

CONCLUSION

Purely hallucinated practice of subordinate-hand writing, under conditions of *time distortion* in hypnosis, gives the subject a feeling of having acquired the practice effects of a similar amount of actual writing in the waking state. Waking performance of tasks practiced as described is accompanied by a feeling of increased ease as compared to pre-practice performance.

There is no evidence, in the results of these experiments, that the learning process itself is facilitated by such practice.

The problem here studied deserves further investigation.

CHAPTER 19

Nonmotor Learning[1]

In the course of our earlier work, reports were occasionally obtained which brought up the possibility that nonmotor learning could be facilitated by trance practice under conditions of time distortion. One subject felt that his learning of poetry was so facilitated. In another case, the subject was having great difficulty learning the stage business in a show which he was rehearsing (2). He was given 6 rehearsal periods, each with an allotted time of 15 seconds and a suggested personal time of 15 minutes, all in one session. The director of the play was not informed as to this practice and, so far as is known, the subject had no further training until the next actual rehearsal. The director, who had been told merely to make special note concerning the subject's performance, stated, when interviewed after the following rehearsal, that "the subject went through his role perfectly." In order to further investigate this possible application of time distortion in hypnosis, the following experiment was performed.

TERMS

In this discussion, presentation time is the time in seconds required to present verbally to the subject the material to be learned. The term "study period" connotes the time allowed the subject for the study of each letter-group-pair, and thus does not include presentation time. Its onset was indicated by the signal "Now", or "Take".

PURPOSE

The purpose of this study was to compare two methods of learning nonsense material. In one, the subject employed certain learning techniques while awake; in the other, he employed the same techniques in

[1] Reprinted, with some changes, from "Time Distortion in Hypnosis and Nonmotor Learning", by Cooper, L. F., and Rodgin, D. W., in Science, 1952, **115**, 500–502.

the hallucinated world, under conditions of time distortion, while in the trance state.

SUBJECT

The subject (I) was a 22-year-old, single, male graduate student in psychology. He was cooperative and intelligent and an excellent hypnotic subject. He had had considerable experience with the experimental use of nonsense syllables, and had been trained in time distortion.

METHOD

Two series of 100 paired nonsense letter-groups of 3 letters each were used. Some of these were syllables; others were consonant groups. Each pair was printed with blue crayon, in large type, on a 3″ x 5″ card thus: CGJ-QXH. The series were of comparable difficulty.

The task was to learn to give correctly, within three seconds, the second group in the pair, in response to the verbal presentation of the first group by the experimenter. At each daily session, five pairs from one series of letter-groups were learned by the subject while awake, and five pairs from the other series while he was in the trance state. Twenty-four hours later he was tested for retention and relearning. Waking and trance tasks were assigned in alternate order on successive days.

1. Learning

At each session there was an initial basic presentation, followed by successive runs through the five cards.

a. Awake: (*1*) *Basic presentation:* The subject sat at a table with pencil and paper at hand, and was instructed to print out each letter-group-pair five times, saying them over to himself and forming associations while doing so. He was to start printing immediately after the presentation of a given pair. The experimenter, in a period of 10 seconds, then read the first pair of letter-groups to him thus: "CGJ, dash, QXH; CGJ, dash, QXH; Now". The "Now" marked the end of the 10 seconds, and was the starting signal for the subject to print the material five times. As he printed, he said the letters to himself and tried to form associations. When this was finished, the pair on the next card was presented in the same way. The average time taken by the printing was 26.5 seconds, making a total average time of 36.5 seconds per letter-group-pair.

(*2*) *Runs:* On completion of the above, the runs were begun, each preceded by a shuffling of the cards. The subject sat with his eyes closed. The experimenter read aloud the first group of one of the pairs, and

TABLE 9

Progress in learning

STUDY PERIOD DESIGNATION	WAKING				TRANCE STATE			
	I (seconds)	II (pairs)	III (pairs)	IV (%)	I (seconds)	II (pairs)	III (pairs)	IV (%)
Basic presentation	26.5	100	38	38	5	100	55	55
First run	5	62	33	53	5	45	35	77
Second run	5	29	22	75	5	10	10	100
Third run	5	7	4	57	5			
Fourth run	5	3	3	100				

I: Avg. duration of study period.

II: Total number of unlearned pairs studied during the 100 study periods of a given designation.

III: Total number of pairs learned in the 100 study periods of a given designation.

IV: Percentage learned of the total unlearned pairs presented during the 100 study periods of a given designation.

the subject immediately stated the second group if he could. At the end of three seconds, the experimenter said, "Take", whereupon the subject opened his eyes and looked at the card. He then immediately closed his eyes and proceeded to memorize during a five-second study period, using non-motor methods. This period was terminated by the presentation of the first letter-group of the next pair. Subsequent runs followed immediately and continued until all the responses were correct. The maximum number of runs required was four.

It is thus evident that a run constituted both a test of performance and an opportunity for learning or for reinforcement.

b. Trance state: A moderately deep trance state was induced by suggestions of sleep.

It is important to point out that the following suggestions and instructions pertain to the subject's experience in the hallucinated world only. This world, incidentally, is very real to him, and it is in this, rather than in the physical one, that he carried out his trance study in distorted time, including the (purely hallucinated) printing. Throughout, he remained motionless, with his eyes closed, except the eye response to "Take".

(1) Basic presentation: The following suggestions were given to the subject:

"You're now going to learn some nonsense letter-groups. You will have ample time between signals to learn them solidly. (This reference to "ample time" was understood by the trained subject to refer to his "special time".) As I give you a pair, you will print it out five times, exactly as you did while awake, saying the letters to yourself and forming associations as you do so. After that you may print them some more, or say the letters over to yourself many times more in order to take advantage of repetition, or form unusual associations, or adopt any other method of learning that you wish. This activity will impress the material upon your memory. It is important that you take as much of your special trance time as is necessary. You will not hurry, and it will be easy to learn them and to recall them later."

During the last 13 sessions the above suggestions were given verbatim. Prior to that, the same ideas were presented, but the wording was varied slightly at times.

Immediately after giving the suggestions, the actual presentation of the material was begun. The subject sat at a table with his eyes closed, and the letter-groups were read to him exactly as in the waking state. Then, at the starting signal, he began his trance study, using distorted time. At the end of only five seconds allotted time, the amount being unknown to the subject, the experimenter gave the termination signal ("Now, blank"), indicating to the subject that he was to stop all mental activity and make his mind a blank. The next pair was then presented. Thus the presentation time was 10 seconds, and the hallucinated activity lasted five seconds.

(2) *Runs:* During the runs, the technique was identical with that used in the waking state, except that the subject, in the five-second study period, closed his eyes again and, using distorted time, practiced much as he had during the basic study period for the trance state.

2. Retention test and relearning

Here the subject was awake throughout. There was of course no basic presentation. Runs were assigned until the responses were all correct. The technique was identical with that already described for runs in the waking state. This testing was generally done 24 hours after the original learning, but in some instances several days intervened.

TABLE 10

Average learning time

AVERAGE LEARNING TIME PER LETTER-GROUP-PAIR	WAKING (SEC.)	TRANCE STATE (SEC.)
Including presentation time......................	41.5	17.7
Not including presentation time..................	31.5	7.7

TABLE 11

Retention and relearning

	AFTER WAKING LEARNING	AFTER TRANCE LEARNING
Retention (%)....................................	19	19
Avg. relearning time per letter-group-pair (sec.)......	6.8	5.1

RESULTS

The subject stated that trance study in distorted time seemed easier than waking study. Not only did he have more time for associations, which in addition came more easily, but he had the benefit of rote practice. He always had plenty of time, and felt that he had really learned the material by the end of the study period, even if he didn't always remember it. He did not hurry, and all activity seemed to him to proceed at the normal or customary rate. Although each study period lasted only five seconds, it seemed to him to be four or five minutes.

DISCUSSION

Under the conditions of this experiment, the results certainly indicate that the study in the trance state was more effective than that in the waking state. Further investigation will be necessary to determine the relative significance, in this facilitation of the learning process, of such factors as post-hypnotic suggestion, increased motivation, and better concentration on the one hand, and of true "utilization" of distorted time on the other. We feel that the latter is of considerable importance, and are inclined to believe that the allotted time could have been cut down from five to three seconds or less without materially altering the results.

SUMMARY

Two methods of learning nonsense material were compared. In one, the subject employed certain learning techniques while awake; in the other, he employed the same techniques in the hallucinated world, under conditions of time distortion, while in the trance state. The average learning time per letter-group-pair, including the time required for presentation of the material, was 41.5 seconds in the former series, and 17.7 in the latter. If the presentation time of 10 seconds is not included, the times are 31.5 seconds and 7.7 seconds, respectively.

Retention was 19 per cent in each series, the average relearning times being 6.8 seconds and 5.1 seconds per letter-group-pair for the waking and trance series, respectively.

Thus the trance study in distorted time was more effective than the waking study.

CHAPTER 20

Mathematical Mental Activity

A large number of experiments were done in order to determine whether distorted time could be "utilized" for the performance of certain types of mathematical mental activity. Different sorts of tasks were employed, among them the following:

1. COUNTING

a. Subject awake

A line of poetry, or a short sentence, was read to the subject by the experimenter. The subject was then to determine the number of letters in the expression. He could do this "in his head", or use pencil and paper. His answer, and the time taken to obtain it, were recorded.

b. Subject in trance state

A similar task was assigned for solution by the subject in his hallucinated world. In some cases, no allotted time was used. In others, a short allotted time, and a relatively long suggested personal time were employed. The answer, and the time taken to obtain it, were recorded.

2. COUNTING

a. Subject awake

A description of the subject's house was obtained, and it was explained to him that the window-panes and the stair steps would be used as "counters" in an imaginary task. A definite order of progression, in counting from pane to pane, window to window, and room to room, was stipulated. A sample waking task follows. "Imagine yourself standing at the second window in the living room, with your finger touching the 3rd pane. When I give you a number to 'count out', you will, in your imagination, proceed from pane to pane, window to window, room to room, in the manner agreed upon. You will touch each pane as you count it, and step on each step as you count it. When you finish, you will tell me at what pane or step you end up. The number is 85—Now." His answer and the time required were recorded.

b. Subject in trance state

Here the phrase, "in your imagination", was omitted. The subject hallucinated the house, of course. A series of tasks were run without an allotted time, and with a short allotted time and a relatively long suggested personal time. The answer and the time involved were recorded.

3. ARITHMETIC

a. Subject awake

Various simple arithmetical problems, or series of simple operations, were assigned. Some of these were to be done "in his head". In others, he could use pencil and paper. The answers and the time were recorded.

b. Subject in trance state

The tasks were similar to those assigned in the waking state. In some cases, no allotted time was used. In others, a short allotted time and a relatively long suggested personal time was employed. In the hallucinated world, the subject did some of the tasks "in his head", some with pencil and paper, some on a blackboard, and, in some cases, he watched a friend do them on a blackboard. The answer and the time were recorded.

4. CODING

a. Subject awake

The numbers from 1 to 26 were assigned, in order, to the 26 letters of the alphabet. These were designated as the code numbers of the letters, and were memorized by the subject. Using these, code numbers for letter-groups, words, or sentences could be obtained in any prescribed fashion, employing stipulated arithmetical operations. Likewise, methods could be prescribed for converting such a number into a letter. Such tasks we refer to as coding tasks, and hundreds of them were used. The waking subject did them "in his head", the answer and the time being recorded.

b. Subject in trance state

The tasks were similar to those assigned in the waking state. In some cases, no allotted time was used. In others, a short allotted time and a relatively long suggested personal time were employed. In performing these tasks in the hallucinated world, the subject did some of them "in his head", some with pencil and paper, some on the blackboard, and in some cases he watched a friend do them on a blackboard. The answer and the time were recorded.

DISCUSSION

Two subjects were used for these experiments, and neither showed any evidence of ability to "utilize" distorted time for the type of mental activity studied. Where no allotted time was used, the subject's performance was approximately the same as in the waking state. Where a short allotted time was used, the performance, in terms of correct answers, was no better than chance would give, even though the suggested personal time was usually accepted in full.

Subject K had difficulty with even the simplest arithmetical problems in the waking state. In the hallucinated solving of the problems, with a short allotted time and a relatively long suggested personal time, she invariably believed that the answer she obtained was correct. Faced with some of her operations, in the waking state, she would reply, "Well, it seemed to be right when I did it." And well it may have, for in our suggestion we always assured the subject that she would not have to hurry, that she would check her work carefully, and that she would get the correct answer.

Subject I, on the other hand, was a good mathematician. His observations on his experience—always unsuccessful—in trying to solve the various problems in distorted time are very revealing. In this sort of task, the action invariably "lacked continuity", or showed "disconnected points". "Thinking of a letter, then getting a number, then adding others, etc.—this is a discontinuous process. You have to shift your operational activity. It doesn't seem to be conducive to promoting or abetting good time distortion."

On the other hand, "Anything that's continuous, such as hand-writing, listening to music, engaging in any sort of continuous activity, and things of that sort, I believe are conducive to producing good time distortion."

Let us compare (a), the hallucinatory counting of a large number of coins as they are removed from a box—an activity that proceeds readily in distorted time and that seems, to the subject, to be "continuous", and (b), the hallucinatory counting, in their order of occurrence, of the letters in a sentence—an activity which invariably seems to be "discontinuous".

In (a), we find the following to be true:

1. The process of counting, per se, as distinct from counting certain objects, is a firmly established pattern.

2. Likewise, the repetitive motor act involved in such a task is a quite familiar one.

3. The production, by the mind, of an hallucinated coin for the hallucinated hand to pick up and place on an hallucinated table is, again, consistent with the well-trained subject's ability.

4. Most important of all—no unknown is involved.

In (b), the following is true:

In counting the letters in a sentence, in the order in which they occur, an association is formed between each letter and a member of a series of unique symbols known as numbers.

In this particular task, the location of the letters in experiential space determines the sequential order in which they are to be associated with a number.

In counting, per se, the individual members of the number series are brought to mind in a definite order or sequence, and the act of counting is extended in experiential time. In counting the letters in our sentence, sequential ordering of the numbers in the number series determines the order in which they are to be associated with a letter.

If we make the association as above stipulated, we shall reach the end of a given line with, let us say, the association between "n" and "36", and can then say that the line contained 36 letters, and that "n" is the 36th in the stipulated order. In other words, we have answered the question, "If we associate the letters with numbers in this stipulated fashion, what number will be associated with the last letter in the line?"

Here, then, the subject is relating the numbers in a stipulated sequence to the letters, likewise taken in a certain sequence. In so doing, each relating of letter to number is a *new* experience.

Whether a waking subject does such a task as the above "in his head", using imagery, or a hypnotized subject hallucinates the process, he must,

1. Know how to count;
2. Remember the sentence and the order in which the letters appear;
3. Associate only one number with each letter, and do this in the stipulated manner.

Apparently, this sort of mental activity cannot proceed, in distorted time, at a rate, relative to world time, that is any greater than in the waking state.

It is interesting to note that any of these operational tasks, if assigned repeatedly, will proceed more and more easily, until finally they become "continuous" and can be completed within a very short allotted time. But when this is achieved, they are no longer problems containing an unknown, but rather are familiar patterns of past experience.

We can say, then, that only those activities which can be constructed from elements of past experience or new combinations thereof, can proceed, in distorted time, at an increased rate relative to world time. The solving of mathematical problems obviously does not fall into this category, for the answer is not to be found in the subject's past experience.

CHAPTER 21

Polygraph Studies

The problem of falsification in reporting was investigated by means of the polygraph, or "lie detector", in a 25-year-old female with a high-school education (subject K). She was the least critically-minded of our subjects. A Keeler polygraph was used, the tests being conducted by a psychologist who had had a wide experience in the use of this instrument. A verbatim report of the experiments, obtained by stenotype, follows.

The letter E stands for the experimenter, S for the subject, and P for the psychologist who conducted the polygraph tests.

EXPERIMENT 1

Polygraph not recording.
Induction of trance state.

1. E. Make yourself comfortable, Miss Jones. You know what we are going to do, don't you? We are going to give you a task and then we are going to ask some questions later, and then we are going to subject you to a polygraph.

Close your eyes, please, and get yourself perfectly comfortable and relaxed. I am going to put you in a deep hypnotic sleep.

You are going deep, deep asleep, into a deep hypnotic sleep, deeper and deeper, deeper and deeper asleep, deep, deep sleep. You are completely comfortable and you are entirely relaxed, and you are going deep asleep, deep asleep, into a deep hypnotic sleep, deeper and deeper, deeper and deeper asleep, deeper and deeper, deeper and deeper asleep, into a deep, deep hypnotic sleep, deep asleep, deep, deep asleep, in a deep hypnotic sleep.

You are now deep asleep, in a deep hypnotic sleep—and in this sleep you will accept and carry out any suggestions that I give to you. Any experiences that you have will be just as real as if you were awake. And you will stay deep asleep until I wake you.

Polygraph not recording.
Subject in trance state.

Now, listen to me carefully, please. When I give you the starting signal by saying "now", you are going to cook a meal. Here comes the signal. Now.

Now blank, please. Your mind is now a blank. Now I am going to wake you by counting to five. When I reach five, you will be wide awake and refreshed and you will remember everything you have done.

One, you are waking, waking, waking. Two, waking, waking, waking. Three, waking, waking, waking. Four, you are almost awake. Five, you are wide awake and refreshed.

Are you awake now, Miss Jones?

2. S. Yes.

Polygraph not recording.

Subject awake.

3. E. Tell me what happened, please.

4. S. Well, I entered the kitchen to prepare dinner, and I had fried chicken. I took the chicken out of the box and salted it and put some pepper on it and flour. I put the pan on the stove, put some grease in it, let it get hot. Then I dropped the chicken in. Then I put a pan on the stove to put some frozen beans in and let the water boil, and while the water was boiling, I peeled some potatoes for french fries and I put the pan on the stove with the potatoes to fry, put some grease in them, and when the grease got hot I dropped the potatoes in the pan, and as I dropped them in, some grease popped on my arm. I burnt my arm, so I put some butter on it right away and the spots began to burn quite a bit. Then it was all right. Then I kept standing over the stove, noticing the chicken. Then I went in the room to sit down and listen to the radio while the food cooked. In about ten minutes it was all ready. I went in and cut the heat off under the chicken and the beans and potatoes.

5. E. Is there anything else?

6. S. No, that's all.

7. E. Was it real?

8. S. Yes, very real.

9. E. How long did it seem?

10. S. About 45 minutes.

11. E. Were there any gaps or omissions?

12. S. None at all.

13. E. Miss Jones, I am going to ask the stenotypist to read back the report that he took down from you—you understand?

14. S. Yes.

(The report was read as requested.)

15. E. You heard it, Miss Jones?

16. S. Yes.

17. E. Was it true or false?

18. S. True.

Polygraph recording.

Subject awake.

19. P. All right. We are ready to begin. Do you now live in Washington?

20. S. Yes.

21. P. Did you go to work today?

22. S. Yes.

23. P. Was the report you gave true?

24. S. Yes.

25. P. Were you born in April?

26. S. Yes.

27. P. Was your trance experience real?

28. S. Yes.

29. P. Have you used your sick leave falsely more than five times?

30. S. No.

31. P. Would you swear to that?

32. S. Yes.

33. P. Have you been on the polygraph before tonight?

34. S. Yes.

35. P. Were there any gaps or omissions in your trance experience tonight?

36. S. No.

37. P. Is today Wednesday?

38. S. Yes.

39. P. Were there any gaps or omissions in your trance experience tonight?

40. S. No.

41. P. Did your trance experience take about 45 minutes?

42. S. Yes.

43. P. Have you falsely answered any of my questions?

44. S. No.

Comment.

The allotted time of the trance task was 10 seconds.

There was no suggested personal time.

The seeming duration of the hallucinatory trance experience was "about 45 minutes".

In the polygraph test, questions 23, 27, 35, 39, 41 and 43 are "relevant" in that they pertain to the trance experience.

Questions 19, 21, 25, 29, 31, 33, and 37 are "non-relevant". Such questions are a necessary part of a polygraph test. They do not pertain to the trance experience.

EXPERIMENT 2

Polygraph not recording.
Induction of trance state.

1. E. You are now relaxing and you are comfortable. You are going deep asleep, into a deep hypnotic sleep. One—deep asleep, deep, deep asleep. Two—you go deeper and deeper, deeper and deeper asleep, into a deep hypnotic sleep. Three—deeper and deeper, deeper and deeper asleep. Four—deep asleep, deeper and deeper, deeper and deeper, into a deep hypnotic sleep. Five—deep asleep, deep, deep asleep. Six—deeper and deeper. Seven—deeper and deeper asleep, into a deep hypnotic sleep. Eight—deeper and deeper, deeper and deeper asleep. Nine—deeper and deeper, deeper and deeper and deeper. Ten—deep, deep asleep, deep, deep asleep.

You are now in a deep hypnotic sleep. And in this sleep, you will be able to accept and carry out any suggestions that I give to you and you will stay deep asleep. And any experiences you have will be very, very real. They will be just as real as if you were awake. But you are going to stay deep asleep until I wake you.

Polygraph not recording.
Subject in trance state.

2. E. Now, give me your attention, please. When I give you the starting signal by saying "Now", you are going to find yourself seated at a table. On that table will be a shoe box full of jelly beans. You will take the jelly beans from the box one at a time and will count them one by one. You will look at each jelly bean as you handle it. You will do this for at least ten minutes. You will not hurry. Is that clear?

3. S. Yes.

4. E. Here comes the starting signal. Now. Now blank. Your mind is now a blank. I am going to wake you now, Miss Jones, by counting to five. When I reach five, you will be wide awake and refreshed.

One—you are waking, waking, waking. Two—waking, waking, waking. Three—waking, waking, waking. Four—you are almost awake. Five—you are wide awake and refreshed.

5. E. Are you awake?

6. S. Yes.

Polygraph not recording.

Subject awake.

7. E. Tell me what happened, please.

8. S. I sat down at the table to count jelly beans, and they were in a large shoe box, all different colors. And I took them out one at a time to count them, and as I counted them, I laid them on the table, and I counted 821 jelly beans.

9. E. Did you look at each jelly bean as you handled it?

10. S. Yes, I did.

11. E. Now, Miss Jones, I would like you to demonstrate for me by counting out loud the rate at which you counted those jelly beans.

12. S. One, two, three, four, five, six, seven, eight, nine, ten, eleven—

13. E. Very good. How long did it seem?

14. S. About ten minutes.

15. E. Did you do anything else?

16. S. No.

Polygraph recording.

Subject awake.

17. P. All right. We are now ready to begin the (polygraph) test, so you just assume the position as usual. Do you have three brothers?

18. S. Yes.

19. P. Do you have two sisters?

20. S. Yes.

21. P. Did you count 821 jelly beans?

22. S. Yes.

23. P. Do you work for Interstate Commerce?

24. S. Yes.

25. P. Did you look at each jelly bean as you handled it?

26. S. Yes.

27. P. Have you ever been drunk?

28. S. No.

29. P. Are you very sure about that?

30. S. Yes.

31. P. Are you now in Washington, D. C.?

32. S. Yes.

33. P. Was your trance experience real?

34. S. Yes.

35. P. Have you ever had your blood pressure taken?

36. S. Yes.

37. P. Were there any gaps or omissions in your experience?

38. S. No.

39. P. Did it seem to take ten minutes?

40. S. Yes.

41. P. Have you falsely answered any of my questions?

42. S. No.

Comment

The allotted time in this experiment was 10 seconds.
The demonstrated rate of counting was 66 per minute.

EXPERIMENT 3

Polygraph recording.
Induction of trance state.

1. E. Are you awake now?

2. S. Yes.

3. E. Close your eyes now, please, and make yourself as comfortable as possible. I am going to put you in a trance again. You are comfortable now and you are relaxed, and you are going into a deep hypnotic sleep. You are going deep, deep asleep, deeper and deeper, deeper and deeper asleep, into a deep hypnotic sleep. Deeper and deeper, deeper, deeper asleep. Are you now in a trance state?

4. S. Yes.

Polygraph recording.
Subject in trance state.

5. E. You are a child. Is that statement true or false?

6. S. False.

7. E. Now, go deeper asleep. Deeper and deeper, deeper and deeper asleep, deeper and deeper, deeper and deeper asleep. You are a child. Is that statement true or false?

8. S. True.

9. E. True. Now, Miss Jones, I am going to wake you by counting to five. When I reach five, you will be wide awake and refreshed and you will remember everything you have done. Here comes a waking count. One—you are waking, waking, waking. Two—waking, waking, waking. Three—waking, waking, waking. Four—you are almost awake. Five— you are wide awake and refreshed.

Polygraph not recording.
Subject awake.

10. E. Are you awake?

11. S. Yes.

12. E. Did you see anything in the trance?

13. S. No.

14. E. Did you hear anything?

15. S. No.

16. E. How did you know you were a child?

17. S. I felt like one. I was four years old—four or five years old. But I didn't see or hear anything.

18. E. Is there anything else?

19. S. No.

EXPERIMENT 4

Polygraph recording.

Induction of trance state.

1. E. Close your eyes now, please. I am going to put you asleep again; you are completely relaxed now and you are comfortable, and you are going into a deep hypnotic sleep. Deep asleep, into a deep, deep hypnotic sleep. Deeper and deeper, deeper and deeper asleep. Deeper and deeper, deeper and deeper asleep. Deep, deep asleep. Are you now in the trance state?

2. S. Yes.

Polygraph recording.

Subject in trance state.

3. E. You are a man. Is that statement true or false?

4. S. False.

5. E. I am going to put you deeper asleep now. Deeper and deeper, deeper and deeper asleep; deeper and deeper, deeper and deeper asleep. You are a man. Is that statement true or false?

6. S. True.

7. E. Now, Miss Jones, listen to me. I am going to wake you by counting to five. When I reach five, you will be wide awake and refreshed and you will remember everything you have done. One—you are waking, waking, waking. Two—waking, waking. Three—waking, waking, waking. Four—you are almost awake. Five—you are wide awake and refreshed.

Polygraph not recording.

Subject awake.

8. E. Did you see or hear anything?

9. S. I could see. I saw myself as a man.

10. E. Did you hear anything?

11. S. No. I didn't hear anything.

12. E. Describe what you saw.

13. S. I could see myself in a man's suit.

POLYGRAPH REPORT

The report from the psychologist who conducted the polygraph tests in the above four experiments follows:

"The opinion of the examiner, based upon these polygrams, is that the subject was telling the truth in her reporting."

DISCUSSION

It should be noted that Experiments 3 and 4 do not involve time distortion. They are presented to illustrate the effect of a deepening of the trance state upon the acceptance of a suggestion.

Thus, in Experiment 3, the suggestion, "You are a child," is not accepted when first given but is accepted after the trance has been deepened. The same is true of the suggestion, "You are a man," in Experiment 4.

It is interesting to note that the subject's acceptance of the suggestion, "You are a child," consists in feeling like a child. Having once been a child, this was a feeling that she had experienced in the past. On the other hand, she had never been a man, and consequently in accepting the suggestion, "You are a man," she could not feel like a man. So instead, she saw herself as a man. Questioned further about this, she said, "It was as if I was seeing myself in a mirror."

CHAPTER 22

A Semantic Interpretation of Verbal Suggestion[1]

The hallucinatory productions in the trance state come, of course, from the unconscious, but we shall not concern ourselves with this aspect of the problem. We shall, rather, consider the *experiential world* of the hypnotized subject—in other words, his present experience, and shall leave to the investigator of the unconscious the depth aspects of the questions treated. The hypnotized subject is keenly conscious and, with some exceptions, his hallucinatory experiences are subject, at least in their broad design, to ego-direction. The use of the word *ego*, in this discussion, is not to be confused with its Freudian use. By *ego* we mean simply, "The conscious and permanent subject of all experience" (Webster).

This treatise, then, considers immediate present experience. After an introductory discussion concerning words, it takes up difference as known in experience, relation, the present, and time. This provides a background for discussing experience from the point of view of its component units. Subsequent sections are devoted to meaning-tone, the semantic significance of the word "is" and the verb *be*, falsification in hypnosis, the quantitation of experience, and finally certain speculations concerning time distortion and the trance state itself.

We shall begin with the following quotation from the book, *Mathematician's Delight*, by Sawyer.

> On the other hand, there are interesting signs of the way in which human thought has been built up through daily experience. One such sign is to be found in the words we use. Try to imagine, if you can, a cave-man (or whoever it was that first developed language) trying to say to a friend, "What

[1] Reprinted, with some changes, from "Time Distortion in Hypnosis, with a Semantic Interpretation of the Mechanism of Certain Hypnotically Induced Phenomena," by Cooper, L. F., in Journal of Psychology, 1952, **34**, 257–284.

this writer says about the square root of minus one does not agree with my philosophy at all." How would he manage to make his friend understand what he meant by such abstract words as "philosophy", "minus one", "agree" and so forth? Every child, in learning to speak, is faced by the same problem. How does it ever come to know the meaning of words, apart from the names of people and objects it can see?

It is instructive to take a dictionary, and to look up such words. Almost always, one finds that abstract words, the names of things which cannot be seen, come from words for actual objects or actions. Take, for instance, the word "understand". Both in German and English it is connected with the words "to stand under". In French, "Do you understand?" is "Comprenez-vous?", which means "Can you take hold of that?" rather like the English phrase, "Can you grasp that?" Still today, people make such remarks as, "Try to get that into your head."

In learning to speak, a child follows much the same road. It learns the names of its parents and of household objects. It also learns words which describe its feelings, "Are you hungry?" "Are you tired?" "He looks happy." "Don't be frightened." "Can't you remember?" "Say you are sorry."

Every philosopher, every professor, every school-teacher that ever lived began in this way—with words to describe things seen, or things felt. *And all the complicated ideas that have ever been thought of, rest upon this foundation.* Every writer or speaker that ever invented a new word had to explain its meaning by means of other words which people already knew and understood. It would be possible to draw a huge figure representing the English language, in which each word was represented as a block, resting on other blocks—the words used to explain it. At the bottom we should have blocks which did not rest on anything. These would be the words which we can understand directly from our own experience—what we see, what we feel, what we do (17).

With the above brief remarks concerning words and their meaning, we shall proceed to discuss certain basic aspects of immediate present experience. Immediate present experience makes up, for each of us, our *experiential world*. This, of course, may include representations of past experience and newly-created combinations of such symbols, the latter including dreams, fantasies, "imaginary" productions, hypotheses, etc. Hallucinations, of course, are a form of present experience. The future, as well as the past and present, can be thought of in such terms.

The space and time of present experience we shall term *experiential space*, and *experiential time*. We can define a point in experiential space as the smallest recognizable "area" of experience ordered in experiential space, and a point in experiential time as the briefest recognizable experience ordered in experiential time.

There is, for each of us, a vast world which we have created from our own past experience, including the communications of others, and from our imagination. Its "contents" are not within our present experience, but are represented therein by ideas, and range all the way from the door in back of me, to the field of awareness which my friend says he experiences, to the electron. In many cases they can be brought into present experience if we are willing to go to the necessary trouble. As a rule, however, we get along quite well by simply assuming that we should find them if we looked, and it is in terms of this world that we plan our daily lives, and our future. This is the *assumptive world*, much of it ordered in *assumptive space*, and all of it ordered in *assumptive time*.

DIFFERENCE

1. Difference as perceived in experiential space

In discussing difference, let us first consider visual experience. Since all visual experience is *extended* in experiential space, we cannot experience difference in quality without difference in extension and in location.

Figure 7 represents two gray circles, A and B, the grayness being identical in quality, intensity, and extension. We shall suppose that their background is a white screen, so placed that the entire field can be perceived at a given instant t. The experience of seeing these circles we shall call E, and the loci of the circles S_1 and S_3 respectively. The area between the circles is locus S_2. E_1 is our experience at S_1 and time t; E_2 is our experience at S_2 and time t; E_3 is our experience at S_3 and time t.

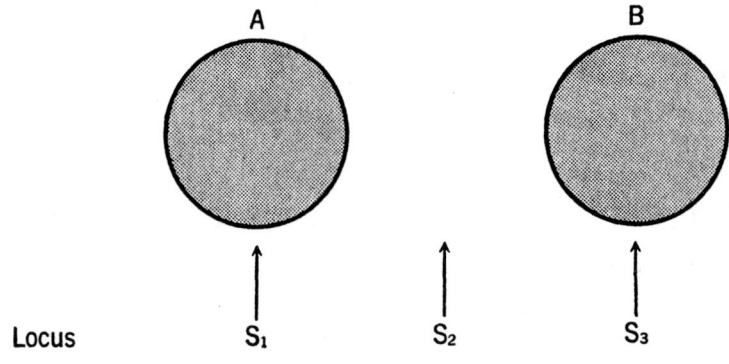

At time t

FIG. 7

The following, then, is true:

(a) E_2 differs from E_1 in quality, intensity, and extension, and locus in experiential space. Of experience E_1, we can affirm, "Grayness is." Of experience E_2, we can affirm, "Grayness is not."

(b) E_3 differs from E_2 in quality, intensity, and extension, and in locus in experiential space. Of experience E_2, we can affirm, "Grayness is not." Of experience E_3, we can affirm, "Grayness is."

(c) E_1 differs from E_3 only in locus in experiential space. Of both E_1 and E_3, we can affirm, "Grayness is."

The following is evident if we consider E_1 and E_2 together:

These experiences are identical in locus in experiential time, but differ in quality, intensity, and extension, and in locus in experiential space.

By these differences, we know the "two-ness" of experiences E_1 and E_2.

At a given locus in experiential time, then, difference in quality or intensity of experience can be known only at different loci in experiential space.

The following is evident if we consider E_1 and E_3 together:

These experiences are identical in locus in experiential time, and in quality, intensity, and extension, but differ in locus in experiential space.

By difference in locus in experiential space alone, then, we know the "two-ness" of experiences E_1 and E_3.

Difference in locus in experiential space, then, is that by which, at a given point in experiential time, we can know "two-ness" in experience that is of uniform quality and intensity.

We can thus say, "Experience is ordered in experiential space if, at time t, 'two-ness' can be known between experiences that are identical in quality and in intensity." We can use this criterion in examining various components of experience.

Two experiences, so knowable as "two", are separated by an interval of experiential space. Since they are experienced at time t, they naturally fall into the present.

2. Difference as perceived in experiential time

Figure 8 represents three sequential experiences at times t_1, t_2, and t_3, respectively, produced by flashing a gray circle, at locus S, twice on a square white screen. The center of the circles coincides with the center of the screen. The circle flashed at t_1 is, of course, identical in grayness and in intensity thereof, and in size, to that flashed at t_3. The flashes each occupy an "experiential instant". The interval between them is 0.06

At time

t_1

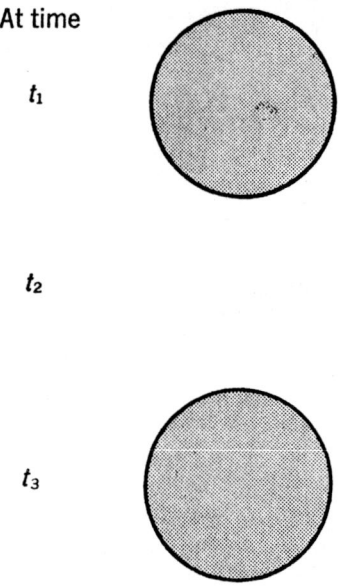

t_2

t_3

At locus S (area on which circle is flashed).

FIG. 8

seconds. Thus the two circles fall within the "duration" of the psychological present.

E_1 is experience at locus S and time t_1 ; E_2 is experience at locus S and time t_2 ; E_3 is experience at locus S and time t_3.

The following, then, is true:

(a) E_2 differs from E_1 in quality and intensity, and in locus in experiential time. Of experience E_1, we can affirm, "Grayness is." Of experience E_2, we can affirm, "Grayness is not."

(b) E_3 differs from E_2 in quality and intensity, and in locus in experiential time. Of experience E_2, we can affirm, "Grayness is not." Of experience E_3, we can affirm, "Grayness is."

(c) E_3 differs from E_1 only in locus in experiential time. Of both E_1 and E_3, we can affirm, "Grayness is."

The following is evident if we consider E_1 and E_2 together:

These experiences are identical in locus in experiential space, but differ in quality and in intensity, and in locus in experiential time.

By these differences, we know the "two-ness" of experiences E_1 and E_2.

At a given locus in experiential space, then, difference in quality or intensity of experience can be known only at different loci in experiential time, i.e., sequentially.

The following is evident if we consider E_1 and E_3 together:

These experiences are identical in locus in experiential space, and in quality, intensity, and extension, but differ in locus in experiential time.

By difference in locus in experiential time alone, then, we know the "two-ness" of experiences E_1 and E_3.

Difference in locus in experiential time (sequence), then, is that by which, at a given locus in experiential space, we can know "two-ness" in experience that is of uniform quality and intensity.

Two experiences, so knowable as "two", are separated by an interval of experiential time. If such an interval is sufficiently brief, the two experiences, and the interval between them, fall into the present, and the interval has a very brief duration therein. Being in the present, memory is not necessary for the appreciation of duration. The experience of longer "durations", or time intervals is, of course, dependent upon memory.

Notice that, in the above example, duration, and sequential difference of experiences, are knowable only in immediate experience, and constitute *experiential time*. Where there is no sequence between two experiences, we say that they are simultaneous. Simultaneity is, like sequence, a relation between two unit experiences, and is known in immediate experience.

It will be remembered that we stipulated that the two flashes in our example were "instantaneous" in that they occupied points in experiential time as defined elsewhere. If we assume this to be true of only one of them, the other still being very brief, we can then say that they are similar in quality, intensity, and extension, and in locus in experiential space, but differ in duration.

In the example in figure 7, we can readily see that our experience was ordered in experiential time, but not extended therein, whereas it was both ordered and extended in experiential space. On the other hand, in the example in figure 8, our experience was both ordered and extended in experiential time (the interval had duration), and ordered and extended in experiential space.

The knowing of difference invariably implies the concomitant knowing of "one-ness" and "two-ness"; of unity and number, and is extremely important.

In the example in figure 7 above, of experience ordered and extended in experiential space at time t, difference in locus in experiential space is known simultaneously with "one-ness", and "two-ness"—as a sort of triad. As mentioned above, difference makes possible the knowing of number.

In the example in figure 8 above, of experience ordered and extended in experiential time, and in experiential space, at a given locus S, we again have the triad, "one-ness", "two-ness", and difference, here in experiential time. Because of the shortness of the time interval, the experience falls into the present. If a longer interval is involved, of course, recall is necessary in order to know sequence.

RELATION

Difference makes possible the experiencing of relation. Relation may be defined as, "any aspect or quality which can be predicated only of two or more things taken together, as direction, resemblance, or of one thing considered as a factor of itself, self-identity" (Webster).

Let us imagine two square blue fields, A and B, each containing two red circles. All the circles are identical in color and in intensity thereof, but those in Field A are arranged vertically, while those in Field B are horizontal. Considering first only Field A, we can affirm that the circles therein are ordered and extended in experiential space. Thus relation exists between them—relation in experiential space. Of the circles in Field B, we can make the same predication. In addition, however, we can say that the spatial relation between the circles in Field A is different from that between those in Field B. The same is true of experience, at time t, that is merely ordered in experiential space, as in the case of two identical sounds.

THE PRESENT

We have seen that some forms of experience come to us extended in experiential space. The fact that several sequential red circles, flashed each for an "instant" upon a white background at very brief intervals, are experienced in the present, demonstrates that the present has duration. In the *present* much experience is extended in both experiential space and experiential time.

It may well be that it is because of the duration of the present that we can recognize occurring change. We say, for instance, "It is changing color," or "It is moving" (changing position in experiential space). When we observe an object moving against its background in our visual field, as it moves, certain portions of the background become sequentially covered and uncovered. It is this, probably, that enables us to discern motion under these conditions. Occasionally, however, we experience motion in an object in the absence of this covering and uncovering. For instance, I have on my desk a glass paper-weight. It has a square base and a spherical dome. If I spin it on its dome and watch it, immediately after it has come to rest it will appear to turn slowly in the opposite direction to the spinning. This illusion is an interesting case of experiential motion, recognized in some other way than that mentioned above.

Let us return, for a moment, to motion as ordinarily perceived in the visual field. We notice that it always has direction, and that this is always away from an earlier position and towards a future one. Thus our appreciation of sequence determines direction. Let us now consider a body that is moving across our visual field, in a straight line. We not only appreciate this fact, but also can tell whether its speed of progress is what we call "constant", or whether it varies. If it varies, we can know whether such change occurs rapidly or slowly. Likewise, if its path be circular, we can know constant or changing speeds along this path. If the path changes direction at random, we can perceive a varying rate of such change. We can say, "It's changing direction rapidly—or slowly." It is, of course, well known that all this is knowable only approximately, and within fairly narrow limits, but, nevertheless, knowable it is, and this is undoubtedly the result of a blend of our appreciation of a body's position in experiential space, relative to other aspects of the field, and of our sense of sequence. In other words, it is due to a blend of our perception of experiential space and of experiential time, occurring in the present—where some experience is extended in experiential space, and some in experiential time, but where most experience is extended in both.

TIME

In our ordinary clock, the series of events provided is the passage of the hands past certain points on the circumference of a circle. Let us consider an electric clock with a long "sweep" second hand, which makes one revolution a minute. The hand thus passes 60 such points in each revolution. As we watch it, we shall note the following: (a) The hand appears to move at a constant rate. (b) The time intervals between its passing of any two successive points seem to be equal. (c) The arcs between such points are equal, being 6 degrees.

Let us now leave consideration of these shorter time intervals and consider the hour hand and the minute hand only. And let us see what we do when, as we are looking at our clock, someone asks the question, "What time is it?"

Simultaneously with this question (simultaneity is known in immediate experience) I note the relative location, in experiential space, of the hands of my clock to the marks on the dial, and say, "It is 12 o'clock."

Now let us repeat this experiment a bit later, and suppose that my answer now is "It is 5 minutes past 12." With this, I am well aware that one reading preceded the other (sequence), and that between the two I have experienced a time interval, which, in this case, had a clock reading of 5 minutes.

I am likely to say, if asked, that the interval was "5 minutes long", for custom sanctions this expression. However, the interval itself has not been measured, and all I can really conclude from my clock reading is that during the interval the clock hand moves over 5 one-minute divisions or through an arc of 30 degrees.

Since we generally use solar time in our measurements, our ordinary clocks indicate to us the relative position between a point on the earth's surface and the sun.

Thus, in effect, our answer to the question, "What time is it?" amounts to saying, "As I note the time, the relation of point P on the earth's surface, to the sun, is this." And, in answering the question, "How long was the interval?" I say, in effect, "During the interval, the point P moved through 1.25 degrees." In one second by our clock such a point would move through 0.00416+ degrees.

Our sense of simultaneity is necessary in order to make a clock reading of any event. The event, in the case of the question "What time is it?" was the question itself, and the reading was taken simultaneously with it. It might just as well have been any other event, such as a pistol shot. Thus, in noting the time at which a pistol shot is heard, we read our clock at that point in experiential time at which we hear the report. In so reading the clock, we note the point on the clock dial at which the moving hand is located at such an instant. If two successive shots are to be timed, the same process is applied in the case of the second shot as in that of the first. Between the two, we experience a sense of duration, and the moving hand changes its locus in experiential space relative to the clock dial and the distance covered can be measured in experiential spatial units. As pointed out previously, however, such units do not in any sense measure our feeling of duration during the interval, for units of change in spatial locus—the seconds used by the physicists and the mathematicians, are a very different thing from experiential time, since they are based upon experiential spatial perception. The failure to realize this has cast much confusion over the problem, "What is time?"

Experiential time is subject to high degrees of distortion. One of the most interesting instances of this is seen, occasionally, in the presence of danger. Many persons have reported that, at such times, movement in experiential space seemed to progress very slowly, and their sense of duration was appropriate to this slowing. Yet an uninvolved observer might state that things happened with great rapidity. This is an instance of that sort of time distortion in which the involved person experiences no more sequential events than does the onlooker, but they seem, to the victim, to proceed very slowly. On the other hand, there are innumerable reports from persons who have nearly drowned and who say that they re-lived great segments of their life, at a normal pace, in what was actually but a few seconds or minutes. Here many sequential events are experienced, in natural tempo, in a very brief interval by the clock. We see a similar phenomenon in the nocturnal dream, and in hallucinated activity under conditions of time distortion in hypnosis. But, alas! there is no onlooker to witness such experiences.

UNITS OF EXPERIENCE, IMAGES, THOUGHT

Experience is heterogeneous, being composed of many parts or groups of parts. There are sensations, drives, feelings, emotions, images, meaning-tone, volition, etc., and memories thereof. Some experience presents what we call intensity, which may vary in degree. Between any two sorts of experience, we can know relation. We can know change. With the aid of memory, we can know and deal with past experience that extended through many "presents". Thus, patterns of experience extended in time, such as a piece of music, or a battle, or any other action, can be appreciated by us. Difference, in short, enables us to perceive experience in units and groups of units.

Among units of primary experience, images and meaning-tone are of special interest to us here. Both are related to past experience, and both are known only through memory.

Images are experiences that resemble portions of past experience, yet are known, by the subject, to differ therefrom in some way. When images simulate such experience so closely as to be undifferentiable therefrom, they cease to be images, as far as the subject is concerned, for to him they have now become "the real thing". Such conviction is characteristic of hallucinatory experience.

It is important to point out that we do not restrict the use of the word "image" to representations of visual experience, but consider it to be applicable to representations of all forms of experience.

There is another form of experience which we refer to as thought. There is probably little to be gained here by entering into the controversy over so-called imageless thought, if for no other reason than that there may be a wide variation, in this regard, between individuals. Suffice it to say that we do think, and that some of us can do a great deal of thinking without employing much imagery or much verbalization. Thus I can prepare a dissertation on "fear", without, to an appreciable degree, experiencing the emotion itself. Or I can think about the impact of the internal combustion engine upon modern culture without carrying the image of such an engine through all my deliberations. Thus, non-verbal thought employs not only images, but something else as well. This other constituent is somewhat akin to a feeling, and we shall call it the *meaning-tone of non-verbal experience*. A given experience apparently enables us later either to recall its image, or to experience a unique sort of feeling which can often be resolved, if we wish, into images. That it cannot always be so resolved is seen in the fact that we often know that we've been places and done things, but are unable to supply details that would have been forthcoming shortly after the event. This feeling (meaning-tone) is different from all other sorts of feeling, just as color is different from sound or taste. More important, however, is the fact that the meaning-tone related to a given experiential unit is different from that related to any other unit, and therefore there are units of meaning-tone corresponding to units of experience. In other words, whereas all units of meaning-tone differ from each other, they still have a quality that is common to all and that permits us to classify them as meaning-tone.

Probably most thought employs images, meaning-tone, and words. Images and meaning-tone make up the class "idea", as this term is commonly used.

MEANING-TONE

All forms of experience have a certain quality in common. It is this quality that permits us to place such different entities as color, sound, touch, taste, odor, feeling, emotion, cognition, volition, etc., in a class designated by the term "experience". This quality is that of being in our field of awareness, and consequently of existing. In other words, what we are aware of exists for us. The knowing of this common mark, that is, the feeling (itself an experience) that what we are aware of has being, is derived from our past, and it constitutes a vague atmosphere in which any given experience is set. We shall call it *experience-tone*. But on having an experience which we have had before, our memory, as a result of former associations, contributes another element to our field of awareness. This element, which makes possible the cognition, recognition, understanding, or meaning of any designated experience, we shall call *meaning-tone*.

Thus, on looking at a familiar object such as a spoon, our visual experience is colored by our entire past experience with spoons. Therefore, in addition to the visual experience, we have a feeling of familiarity or of recognition. In other words, the spoon *means* something to us. Meaning-tone that is aroused by non-verbal experience we call the *meaning-tone of non-verbal experience*.

Now let us consider a child who has not yet learned to talk, but who is familiar with spoons. Every time he sees a spoon he will also experience the associated meaning-tone. Now suppose that someone points to a spoon that the child sees and says "spoon". An association is then formed in the child's mind between the visual experience of seeing a spoon and the auditory experience of hearing the word "spoon"—and in the future the hearing of the word will arouse the same meaning-tone that hitherto was aroused on seeing a spoon. Meaning-tone that is aroused by verbal experience we call the *meaning-tone of verbal experience*. It corresponds roughly to the connotation of the word, in the sense that a word "connotes the very various and subtle thoughts and emotions which cluster about that idea in the human mind" (Barrett Wendell). In logic this is referred to as "meaning in intension". We use the term "meaning-tone" in preference to "meaning" alone in order to emphasize the fact that it refers to a feeling, just as do the words recognition, belief, curiosity, doubt, etc., and, as in their case, it is a qualitatively unique feeling. In hearing a sentence which we understand, we *feel* the meaning. A good reader, who does not verbalize, will experience at a glance the meaning-tone of large groups of words. In so doing, we may say that he experiences the *idea* expressed by such words. Thus, what we refer to as the meaning-tone of a verbal experience is, in most ways, similar to what we refer to as the meaning-tone of non-verbal experience, and, like it, is divisible into units. An idea, then, is a unit of meaning-tone, non-verbal or verbal, and/or of imagery. Every word which we understand is capable of arousing in us one or more units of meaning-tone, depending upon the number of definitions it has. These units of meaning-tone, or ideas, have a unique property in that they are resolvable into other units of meaning-tone, and into images of previous experience. In other words, they are resolvable into the units of which they are composed.

The following examples will aid us in isolating meaning-tone for study:

(a) Let us suppose that someone says for us a word in a foreign language which we don't understand. We perceive the sound of the word, of course. And we have a feeling of hearing something we don't understand, possibly along with one of curiosity. Now let the person explain the meaning of the word to us. The next time he says the word, we shall have an entirely different feeling when we hear it. It will mean something to us. It will have conveyed to us an idea.

(b) Many persons have noticed that, if they say a word over and over again, with their attention focussed upon the sound of the word, it loses its meaning temporarily, and a familiar word seems to be nonsense. Here the meaning-tone becomes lost.

(c) We have all had the experience of having an idea and yet being unable to express it. Under such circumstances, we may say, "I know (i.e., feel) what I want to say, but I can't put it into words." This is an example of pre-verbalization meaning-tone.

We can make clear what we mean by the *resolution* of meaning-tone if we consider what we do when someone asks us to explain to him the meaning of a word which he doesn't understand. The word at once arouses in us a unit of meaning-tone, that is, an idea. As we attend this, other units of meaning-tone, which we may or may not verbalize, as well as certain images, take its place. If we continue this process long enough, all the units of meaning-tone are finally resolved to their component images of primary experience. We can verbalize aloud from time to time, until our friend says that he understands.

All meaning-tone, therefore, is resolvable to images, and it can all be communicated, by words, to another person. The images likewise can be verbalized, but unless the other person has had the experience to which the words refer, he can never experience it solely as the result of hearing the words.

It is quite obvious from the above that meaning-tone depends upon past experience. But the most important thing about it is that it is a form of feeling that is unique both qualitatively and in that it is resolvable in the manner described.

Although meaning-tone itself is a part of our immediate present experience, it depends upon memory, just as images do. The following classification of present experience may prove useful to the reader, for it shows the relation of meaning-tone to other concepts that are of importance in the ensuing discussion.

Present experience
Type I
Experience that is not dependent upon memory
(a) Non-verbal
(b) Verbal
Type II
Experience that is dependent upon memory
(a) Imagery
(b) Meaning-tone

AFFIRMATIONS, AND THE VERB "BE"

A child, learning to talk, repeatedly hears affirmations made by others about his immediate present experience. Many such affirmations, moreover, are made concerning a specifically designated portion of his experience with the intention, on the part of an older person, of forming an association in the child's mind between such a portion of his experience and certain verbal symbols. This may be done in response to a question by the child, who may merely point inquiringly to an object such as a book, or who may point to it and ask "What's that?" On the other hand, his elder may draw the child's attention to a book by pointing to it and saying, "Book", or, "That is a book."

In the above process, the child's attention is focussed upon a designated entity (or experiential unit) within his field of awareness. At the same time, of course, he experiences whatever meaning-tone may be associated with this non-verbal experience. Simultaneously with these events, he has the auditory experience of hearing a group of sounds. In the specific instance mentioned above, then, the following elements share the child's field of awareness:

(a) Seeing a book (a type I experience).
(b) The meaning-tone of the book which he sees (a type II experience).
(c) Hearing the words, "That is a book" (a type I experience).

Because of this close association between (a), (b), and (c) we would expect that, in the future, the presence in experience of any one of these three elements would tend to bring the other two to mind.

Let us now suppose that the child later hears a person in another room say, "This is a book." This will arouse in his mind meaning-tone similar to (b) above and he may experience a vague image of a book. Thus the words now have meaning to him, although he himself sees no book. Likewise, in the future, seeing a book will arouse meaning-tone and he can verbalize this by saying, "This is a book."

In the hypnotized subject, a verbal affirmation concerning his experience not only arouses its meaning-tone, but this meaning-tone may cause the subject to have the non-verbal experience with which it has been associated in the past. Thus, if we point to a package of cigarettes that the subject sees and say, "This is a book," he will have the experience of seeing a book rather than a package of cigarettes. While learning to talk, he always saw a book as he heard the affirmation "This is a book," and this may have some bearing on the fact that he hallucinates such an experience later when the affirmation is made to him in the trance state. Thus, the hearing of the verbal affirmation arouses the associated meaning-tone and this in turn leads to an hallucinatory type II experience. This experience resembles those which in the past have been associated with this meaning-tone. Such hallucinatory experiences truly exist or have being for the subject. In other words, for him they are very "real".

It goes without saying that a child hears countless affirmations concerning designated portions of his immediate present experience. The great majority of these contain the verb "be", in the present tense, thus: "Kitty is purring." "The dog is chasing the ball." "They are big boys." "You are tall." Of the three forms of the present tense of be—"am", "are", "is"—the last is probably most often heard. In any event, many many affirmations using many different words are heard, but the words "is", "are", and "am" occur far more often than any others. Now if we bear in mind that these affirmations usually refer to designated portions of the child's immediate present experience, it is easy to see that the verb be becomes associated with experience. And, since what we are aware of exists for us, it comes to be associated with the existence of things. This will be brought out by paraphrasing a few affirmations as follows:

(1) Kitty is purring. I am aware of a purring kitty. A purring kitty exists (for me).

(2) The dog is chasing the ball. I am aware of a dog chasing the ball. A dog chasing the ball exists (for me).

(3) They are big boys. I am aware of those big boys. Those big boys exist (for me).

(4) You are tall. I am aware of a tall you. A tall you exists (for me).

The verb be then comes to have an existential meaning, or usage. Employing the verb in this sense, the simplest thought that I can have concerning experience is the affirmation, "It is." When I say this, I mean "It exists." I don't mean that I think it exists, that I wonder if it exists, that I doubt if it exists, or that I assume that it exists. Nor does my affirmation infer any verbal symbolization of what I experience. I simply mean than I am aware of experience to which I refer by the pronoun "it", i.e., that for me my experience has being, or "isness". I am aware of it, "It is."

In the above discussion, the use of the word "it" implies that I differentiate experience from the experiencer of all experience—the ego-subject from the nonego. This ego-subject is named "I". And when I say "It is," I know it exists; I am convinced of the truth of the affirmation. This conviction is a feeling—a feeling akin to belief, and it is born of experience. I may affirm then, what is a truism, "What I am aware of, is." It is most important to point out that, as I make this affirmation, I have a feeling of belief or conviction. Evidence of the close relation between other experience and belief is found in the old proverb, "Seeing is Believing."

We hope that our interpretation of the affirmation "It is," now has meaning for the reader. This use of "is" here is the same as that of "am" in the affirmation, "I am." And, we repeat, it implies the completion of the ego-nonego differentiation, for without experience there can be no experiencer. It also implies a philosophical turn of mind on the part of the affirmer.

It will be noted that "is", in the above affirmations, is not used in the so-called "copulative" sense, as it does not indicate a relation between subject and predicate.

Let us now examine the use of the word in this latter way, by considering the sentence, "An apple is a fruit." Here "is" obviously indicates a relation between the concept "apple" and the concept "fruit", this relation being that of part to whole. In resolving the meaning-tone of this sentence, we shall resolve that of the two concepts in turn. In this process, at some point, we shall be aware of certain "units" that are present in both concepts. If we consider such units of meaning-tone, and/or images, we can, with the aid of recall, affirm of them, "These from 'apple' are similar to these from 'fruit'." Or, "This group of units from 'apple' is similar to this group of units from 'fruit'." In so affirming we are using "is" in its existential sense.

Again, in the sentence, "The only person in view is my brother", in resolving the meaning-tone of the phrase "The only person in view", on the one hand, and of "my brother" on the other, we find a common experiential unit. This unit is the image of my brother, and the relation is one of identity.

Analysis will reveal the same meaning to "is" in its use in syllogistic reasoning. It merely consists of affirming a similarity or a difference—relations that are knowable in immediate experience—between two primary units of present experience. Though a copulative, its existential sense is retained.

But the word "is" (and the verb be) is not always used in the existential sense. Suppose, for instance, that I come across a strange object, and examine it carefully, finding out a good deal about it in the process. Later I see some people putting it to use, and my information concerning the object is further increased. With all this knowledge, I can do a good deal of thinking about it, even though I don't know its name.

Now let us suppose that someone comes along, points to the object in my presence, and says, "Bazooka".

My experience thereupon may be described as follows. I see the man pointing to the object, and I hear him say, "Bazooka". This forms an association in my mind between the object pointed to and a certain sound. Consequently, in the future, the sound will arouse in me the meaning-tone of the object, and possibly an image of it.

In this pointing to things and naming them, the person so doing usually says, "This is a bazooka (or other name)." Or, in naming a past or future experience, he might use the sentence, "That was a bazooka," or, "That will be a bazooka." Thus the word "is" and the verb *be* come to have, in addition to the existential meaning-tone, the meaning-tone associated with "pointing to", or indicating, an object. We shall call this the *symbol-fixing* meaning-tone of the word "is" and the verb *be*. So we see that, in the above instance, object and name are linked by a verbal experience (the word "is", or some form of the verb *be*), which has *two meanings*, i.e., conviction of existence on the one hand, and a "pointing to" on the other.

Thus, while looking at a book, we can now say, (*a*) "It is." This is equivalent to saying, "That thing (the book) exists." (*b*) "It is a book." This is equivalent to saying, "That thing is called a book."

In brief, then, whenever the verb *be* is heard or read, in its meaning-tone *both* of the above components occur. This fact is of great importance in the mechanism of response to suggestion in the trance state, for it provides the link between the spoken word and non-verbal experience, since all affirmations in the present tense can be re-stated in a form in which the verb *be* appears. The meaning-tone of a given verbal affirmation is thus associated with the visual or auditory perception of the words through the symbol-fixing use of the verb *be*, and with non-verbal experience through its existential use. As will be seen below, in the trance state, a suggestion arouses first this dual meaning-tone, by virtue of the symbol-fixing association, and then this meaning-tone gives rise to the experience from which its existential component was built up.

Now let us imagine that an adult is instructed to respond to my statement to him, "You are a child," by saying, "I am a child." Even though he is wide awake and knows this to be false, the mere saying of the sentence must call forth in him, in meaning-tone, a vague and tenuous *feeling* of conviction that he is a child, although he knows only too well that he isn't. And if we ask him whether the statement is true or false, he will reply, "False".

Now let us hypnotize him, and repeat the experiment. After hearing our statement, he will repeat it in the first person. His experience, thereupon or shortly thereafter, will depend upon how good a subject he is, as well as upon our own technique. There are three possibilities:

(*a*) It may be identical to that in the waking state, and when asked about the truth of the statement, he will say, "False".

(*b*) He may experience the conviction that he is a child and, when asked, tell us that the statement is true. There may be no other hallucinated activity of any sort. If we ask him how he knows he's a child, he may say, "I just know it, that's all." He "knows" it because he believes it. To him, the affirmation is true. He is accurately verbalizing his meaning-tone.

(*c*) He may have the experience described in (*b*) plus varying degrees of hallucinated activity, such as playing with his toys, talking to his parents, etc. In any event, such hallucinated activity will be appropriate to, and supportive of, the affirmation and the accompanying belief to the effect that he is a child. So, when asked, he will reply to us that the statement is true. And if we ask him how he knows that he is a child, he might say, "Because I was playing with my toys."

Of course, the above trance experience could have been produced without his verbally responding to my suggestion, "You are a child," by saying, "I am a child."

From the above we see that in hypnotic suggestion we reverse the process seen in verbalization, i.e., a specific experience → meaning-tone → word, so that it becomes, word → meaning-tone → specified experience. And thus, by means of words, we actually *give* experience. This, we believe, is the basic mechanism involved in the response to suggestion in the trance state.

Time distortion in hypnosis is effected in exactly the same way. Here we can give to the subject great amounts of experience, in the form of sequential events, if we wish, and all with an appropriate sense of the passage of time. Or, by direct suggestion, he can experience duration per se.

FALSIFICATION

Before considering falsification, we wish to call attention to a few of the properties of sentences. A sentence may indicate an affirmation, an interrogation, or a demand, and its meaning-tone will include the corresponding feeling, i.e., something resembling conviction, doubt, or insistence. These feelings are communicated by the words themselves, their order, and the way in which they are said. Interrogation is conveyed usually in all three of these ways in auditory verbalization, and by a question-mark when written. However, in speaking, interrogation may be expressed solely by inflection. Likewise, a spoken affirmation may convey greater or less conviction, depending upon the stress placed upon certain words. Incidentally, inflection, timing, and emphasis, are factors of great importance in hypnotic suggestion.

We have already pointed out that in every affirmation there is the element of belief. This element, which is found invariably, we shall call *affirmation-tone.*

In the second of the three possible reactions to the affirmative suggestion listed above, only a deep conviction of the truth of the statement was experienced by the subject. In other words, in the trance state, the suggestion led the subject to believe the affirmation, but not to produce confirmatory hallucinatory experience. Yet the absence of such hallucinatory experience does not indicate that the subject was falsifying.

In the third possible reaction listed, on the other hand, both belief and confirmatory hallucinatory experience were present. This supportive activity may proceed all the way to a detailed image-production. Or it may stop short of this, or it may be "spotty"—incomplete in regard to some concepts, but complete in regard to others. It certainly can never be complete where the suggested material, or parts thereof, mean nothing to the subject in terms of experience. An honest subject may, under these circumstances, do one of several things, of which the following two are samples. He may simply report no hallucinatory experience. Or he may "hide" the unknown entity in something familiar. Thus, one of our subjects, told that he would see a "bremfra", reported seeing a woman carrying a parcel. In the parcel was the "bremfra".

It is to be emphasized that the failure of a subject to report supportive or confirmatory hallucinatory experience in no way implies that he is falsifying. Naïve observers are only too prone to jump to the wrong conclusion in this regard. One of our subjects reported, after a few seconds of hallucinated activity, that she was sitting with a group that was discussing the meaning of a certain quotation. This is exactly what had been suggested to her. On inquiry as to what they had said, she replied that they had said that "justice is good", this being nothing more than the obvious meaning of the quotation. Questioned further, she insisted that she heard and understood every word. Upon our pointing out that this was a very meager report on a conversation that she said lasted 20 minutes, we were again disappointed by her merely paraphrasing what she had already said. Now, on the face of it, this looks like falsification.

So let us consider a hypothetical waking situation. Mr. *A* meets Mrs. *B* on the street. They stop and talk for 10 minutes about a certain presidential candidate *C*. Mr. *A* is rather impatient, and rather bored, and very much out-talked by the woman, who chatters on at great length.

Soon thereafter, I meet Mr. *A*, who tells me about his encounter. Then I ask him some questions:

> *Q*. What did she have on?
> *A*. I don't know. I didn't notice.
> *Q*. But she had something on, didn't she?
> *A*. I hope so. Yes, of course she did.
> *Q*. How long did she talk to you?
> *A*. Too long. Maybe 10 minutes. Maybe 20.
> *Q*. What did she talk about?
> *A*. About candidate *C*.
> *Q*. What did she say about him?
> *A*. She hopes he gets beaten in the election.
> *Q*. What else?
> *A*. That was the gist of what she said.
> *Q*. Nothing more?
> *A*. She talked a lot, but that was about all she said.
> *Q*. And you mean to say that you listened to her for 10 minutes?
> *A*. At least.
> *Q*. Did you hear and understand every word?
> *A*. Of course I did. But I didn't pay enough attention to remember it all.

No one would think that Mr. *A* was falsifying in any way. He forgot the meaning-tone of many of Mrs *B*'s sentences, though he certainly heard every word. And, what's more important, he remembered, in a sense, what she said.

This is very similar to our subject's report. The difference lies in the fact that the gaps in Mr. *A*'s report were due to lack of attention, or to forgetting the "supporting evidence". In our subject's report, on the other hand, the gaps were the result of the fact that she herself had no ideas on the quotation other than the meager report she gave of the conversation.

Both Mr. *A* and our subject *knew* that they had had the experience they reported. In the case of the subject, she knew it through *belief*, having accepted the affirmation contained in the suggestion, plus such concomitant hallucinatory activity as she produced. When one states what one knows to be true, we don't consider it falsification.

There are undoubtedly many factors which determine the amount of supportive hallucinatory activity. It will vary according to whether the subject is to relive a past experience or to create a new one—whether the activity is a familiar one or not—whether it is simple or complex. The subject's personality make-up, his attitude toward the task, the wording of the suggestion, and the depth of the trance are likewise important. Finally, there are those factors which determine the release of material from the unconscious. One thing is certain—hallucinations can be constructed only from "units" which one has known in past experience.

EXPERIMENTS

As a prelude to presenting the experiment reports, it is advisable to offer the following classifications:

Our discussion of meaning-tone enables us to delineate three stages in its resolution, as follows: *Primary stage*, No resolution; *Secondary stage*, Partial resolution into component units and/or images; *Tertiary stage*, Complete resolution into images. In a somewhat similar fashion, we can consider the possible types of response to the affirmation, *as a whole*, expressed in any suggestion. These are:

(*a*) *Negative response.* The subject's response is similar to that produced by the suggestion when given in the waking state. (*b*) *Primary response.* There is the experience of *believing* the affirmation to be true, but no supportive hallucinatory activity. (*c*) *Secondary response.* There is not only belief in the truth of the affirmation (primary response), but varying degrees of supportive hallucinatory activity as well. In some of the component units of the affirmation, however, there may be either a negative, or a primary, response only. We may, if we wish, speak of "early" or "advanced" secondary responses. (*d*) *Tertiary response.* In addition to a primary response to the affirmation as a whole, there is a rich supportive hallucinatory production comparable, in detail, to waking experience.

This classification permits us to analyze our subject's response to a given suggested affirmation, or, as will be done below, to the component parts thereof. In the latter case, of course, each of these parts is considered to be a "whole" in itself.

In the experiments reported here the allotted time was one second. The first two are reported verbatim. The letter E stands for experimenter, S for subject.

EXPERIMENT 1

1.* E. When I give you the starting signal by saying "Now", you will hear someone recite the first verse of a familiar poem. Now.—Now blank.

2. E. Tell me what happened, please.

3. S. I heard someone recite 4 lines of "The Honest Man".

4.* E. At the next signal, you're going to hear a verse from a Lithuanian poem. Now.—Now blank.

5. E. Tell me what happened, please.

6. S. I heard someone reciting 4 lines from a piece of poetry.

7. E. What language was it in?

8. S. English.

9. E. Did you understand it?

10. S. No.

11. E. Why?

12. S. The words weren't distinct enough.

13.* E. At the next signal, you're going to hear another verse from a Lithuanian poem in Lithuanian. Now.—Now blank.

14. E. Tell me what happened, please.

15. S. I heard a man's voice reciting a piece of poetry.

16. E. Anything else?

17. S. I couldn't understand it.

18. E. Can you repeat any of it?

19. S. No.

20.* E. At the next signal, you're going to hear a Lithuanian woman tell about going to market, in Lithuanian. Now.—Now blank.

21. E. Tell me what happened, please.

22. S. I heard a lady's voice talking, and she was speaking very fast. I couldn't understand her.

23.* E. At the next signal, you're going to hear a Lithuanian woman tell about going to market, in Lithuanian, *and you will understand what she's saying.* Now.—Now blank.

24. E. Tell me what happened, please.

25. S. I heard a lady telling me about her trip to the market.

26. E. Anything else?

27. S. I understood what she was saying.

28. E. Can you tell me about it?

29. S. She was telling about the nice vegetables she had from the

* Asterisk indicates a direct suggestion.

market, how the greens were nice and fresh, and how crowded the market was. (Subject was here stopped from further reporting.)

30. E. What language did she speak?
31. S. It wasn't English.
32. E. Are you sure you understood her?
33. S. Yes.
34. E. What language was it, do you know?
35. S. No.
36. E. Was it Lithuanian?
37. S. I don't know.
38. E. Was it a language you understood?
39. S. I understood what she was saying.
40. E. Did you know the language?
41. S. No.
42. E. How, then, could you understand?
43. S. I don't know, but I did.

At this point, the subject was waked.

44. E. Do you have anything to say about this?
45. S. I could hear her talking, and all. I understood what she was saying, but I don't know what language she was using.
46. E. Did you understand me to say Lithuanian?
47. S. Yes.
48. E. Have you ever heard the word before?
49. S. No.
50. E. Say it for me.
51. S. I can't pronounce it.
52. E. Was the experience real?
53. S. Yes.

In analyzing these reports for supportive hallucinatory activity, let us remember that we must look for a response that is more than a mere reaffirmation or paraphrasing of the original suggestion.

Response to Suggestion 1. In 2 and 3, we see that this is a tertiary response. The subject heard four lines from a certain poem that she had memorized some time previously.

Response to Suggestion 4. This is probably an early secondary response. As seen in 46–51, she had never heard, and couldn't even pronounce, the word "Lithuanian", which probably meant to her merely a strange language. Answer 8, "English", is therefore somewhat of a surprise until it occurs to us that Lithuanian poems are translated into English. Never having heard a Lithuanian poem in any language, she could not produce anything understandable, 9 and 10. So, as seen in 11 and 12, what she heard was indistinct. It is a not uncommon experience to overhear indistinct conversations and yet be fairly certain that they are in English.

Response to Suggestion 13. In view of the evidence, in the subject's previous report, of the resourcefulness of the unconscious, we worded 13 in such a way as to corner her. The response is a primary one, 14 through 19.

Response to Suggestion 20. Here, while still suggesting that she hear Lithuanian, we assigned more readily producible material as the topic. The response, as seen in 21 and 22, is early secondary, for "She was speaking very fast." That the response to the word "Lithuanian" in suggestions 13 and 20 was negative is seen in 36 and 37.

Response to Suggestion 23. Suggestion 23 is the same as 20 except that the additional suggestion, "You will understand what she's saying," was given explicitly and emphatically.

The subject's response is a secondary one, as seen in 24 and 25, 28 and 29, 44 and 45. Note that she insists that she understood, 26 and 27, 32 and 33, and produced supportive hallucinatory activity in the form of hearing a woman talking, as well as supportive meaning-tone. In 50 and 51 is seen her inability to pronounce the word "Lithuanian". In 38 and 39, she herself spontaneously reveals that she experienced the meaning-tone of the woman's words, although she didn't know her language, 40 and 41, 44 and 45. In 42 and 43, she sticks by her guns, and offers no explanations.

Incidentally, it may well be that some nocturnal dreams consist largely of meaning-tone, with relatively little visual or auditory hallucination. In our work on time distortion in hypnosis, however, we are interested in obtaining productions that are "very real" in respect to such hallucinatory activity.

In neither the above nor the following experiment did we inquire concerning visual hallucinatory activity.

EXPERIMENT 2

1.* E. When I give you the starting signal, by saying "Now", you will hear a man discuss Schoenlein's disease. Now.—Now blank.

E. Now tell me about it please.

2. S. I heard a man discuss Schoenlein's disease.

3. E. Did you understand the words?

* Asterisk indicates a direct suggestion.

4. S. No.

5. E. Did you hear the words?

6. S. Yes.

7. E. Were they words you knew?

8. S. Yes.

9. E. Did you understand them?

10. S. No.

11.* E. At the next signal, you will hear a man discuss Schoenlein's disease, and you will understand what he says. Now.—Now blank.

E. Now tell me what happened.

12. S. I heard a man discussing Schoenlein's disease.

13. E. Anything else?

14. S. And I understood what he was saying.

15. E. Tell me what he said.

16. S. (Pause)—(E. urged S. to answer). I can't explain it.

17. E. Are you sure you understood?

18. S. Yes.

19. E. Why can't you explain it then?

20. S. I can't explain it like he explained it to me.

21. E. Explain it to me in your own words, then.

22. S. I can't. I just understand it.

23. E. Are you sure you understand it?

24. S. Yes.

25. E. Positive?

26. S. Yes.

At this point the subject was waked.

27. E. Anything to say?

28. S. I don't like them because I can't tell you what happened. I could hear him talking and I understood—I even understood what he was saying, but I can't explain it.

29. E. Are you sure you understood?

30. S. Yes.

31. E. Is there any question in your mind about that?

32. S. No.

33. E. Do you know anything about Schoenlein's disease?

34. S. No.

35. E. Did you ever hear the word before?

36. S. No.

37. E. Did you hear every word?

38. S. Yes. I just got a general idea of the disease he was discussing.

39. E. Can you tell it to me?

40. S. No.

41. E. Why not?

42. S. I just can't explain it the way he explained it.

43. E. Can you explain it in any other way?

44. S. No. I just understood what he was saying.

We shall not comment in detail upon experiment 2, further than to point out the "solidity" of conviction shown in the primary response to the affirmation "and you will understand what he says," in 11. It can readily be interpreted in greater detail by the reader, in the manner exemplified in the first one. It is interesting to note, however, that in 28 we see evidence of the desire, on the part of a good subject, to carry out a suggestion completely. Here the subject's production, because the term "Schoenlein's disease" meant very little to her, was very meager, and this gave her a feeling of frustration.

EXPERIMENT 3

1.* E. When I give you the starting signal by saying "Now", you will see a little girl. You will pay special attention to what she is wearing, so that you can tell me about it. Now.—Now blank.

E. Tell me about it please.

2. S. (The subject gave a very detailed description of a child who was waiting for a bus. She had on a blue gingham dress, with red trimmings, a necklace, and patent leather shoes.)

3. E. What did she look like?

4. S. (Subject stated that she was about 11 years old, and described her hair and features.)

5. E. Have you ever seen the child before?

6. S. No.

Experiment 3 illustrates the richness of the response when a highly meaningful task was assigned.

We have had literally scores of this type of report in our studies of time distortion in hypnosis, and generally interrupt them in order to get along with the work. Subjects are as likely to create new combinations out of familiar smaller units of experience, as was the case above, as they are to produce entire scenes or actions that they have actually experienced in the past. This can be controlled, of course, by direct suggestion, and this fact raises the possibility that creative thinking might be subject to facilitation by this technique.

* Asterisk indicates a direct suggestion.

We hope that we have shown, by now, that all that appears to be falsification is not such. In fact, when dealing with an honest subject, so-called retrospective falsification or elaboration, in reporting experience, may well be rare. We need hardly point out that, when a subject reports his experience of conviction, we do not consider such reporting to be falsification. In so doing, he is truthfully and accurately reporting on his immediate present experience. It would seem quite obvious, then, that for accurate experimental work, the *sine qua non* is to deal only with intrinsically honest individuals. If this is done, and reports are analyzed as shown above, there may be removed from hypnosis the stigma that now surrounds it in many persons' minds, and that expresses the assumption, by many, that most of the phenomena are the result of an attempt on the part of the subject, be it deliberate or unconsciously motivated, to deceive the experimenter. Due to this attitude, phenomena that may well prove to be of great importance in the understanding of mind, are viewed, with "jaundiced eye" and tongue in cheek, as being evidence of some form of trickery.

THE QUANTITATION OF EXPERIENCE

As work with time distortion in hypnosis has progressed, less and less use has been made of the production, by direct suggestion, of intervals of experiential time (suggested personal time), and we have come to place more emphasis on the production of a series of events, each extended in experiential time. These proceed at a normal or customary rate as far as the subject is concerned, and his experiential time is appropriate. Such an event may consist of anything from a simple action, such as removing a coin from a box and placing it on a table, to such activities as hearing a piece of music, watching a movie short, or playing a game of tennis. The value of such units of action is that they can be counted. This gives us a method of quantitating experience, and of controlling it in quantitative, as well as qualitative, terms. For instance, we assume that, in a given allotted time of, say, one second, a subject would experience a greater number of hallucinatory events in removing from a box and placing on a table 500 coins, than in doing the same with 100. It also provides us with a sort of "subjective clock", since it supplies us with a series of events which can be counted. Since these hallucinated activities are remembered, we naturally assume that they make some sort of impress upon the central nervous system, and are probably accompanied by electrical activity. This at once raises the question as to whether, by producing a large number of sequential hallucinated events in a very brief interval as measured by a stop-watch, properly placed intracerebral electrodes might not show evidence of such electrical activity, which would vary with the "amount" of experience.

MISCELLANEOUS CONSIDERATIONS

It may well be that the infant is unaware of an ego-nonego difference. If so, at this period there can be, for him, only experience (without an experiencer), qualitatively heterogeneous, and increasingly so as sequential events follow one another. Through vision, at least, he early knows experiential space, and motion therein, and his random movements bring much new experience to him, while memory makes possible ideation, and he eventually finds that he can voluntarily change his experience through movement. It is here, possibly, that he first becomes aware of the ego-subject.

Since directed thought, at this period in development, is probably very limited, we can assume that volition is pretty well confined to changing the spatial relations of that large segment of his experience that is ordered in experiential space, and which will later come to constitute, for him, the "physical" world. In fact, the only way in which he can change this portion of his experience is to move its component units. Indeed, in the last analysis, man's progress in "conquering" nature, whether it be exemplified by the building of a great dam, or by the effecting of nuclear fission, has been made solely by rearranging, in experiential space, certain portions of his experience that are *ordered* therein.

Eventually our erstwhile infant has not only made the ego-nonego differentiation, but he divides experience into what he calls a "physical" world, of which his body is a unique part, and a "subjective" world. He is likely to forget that both are still experience. Every time he moves a finger or picks up an object he is merely changing the pattern of that form of experience that is ordered in experiential space, just as, in directed thought, he is changing the pattern of another segment of his experience. And although his thoughts, his feelings, or his dreams, are different from the grayness, coldness, and resistance to his moving hand that go to make up the stone wall that he examines, still, all are experience, all can be recalled, and all can be hallucinated.

The ego-nonego relation is a most baffling one. Its parts are different, yet inseparable. We can focus our attention upon any segment of our experience, from the view we gaze upon to our innermost thoughts and feelings, but the elusive experiencer—the ego-subject, can never be "caught". Since the ego seems to have been derived from experience itself, possibly we should consider seriously Prospero's declaration that, "We are such stuff as dreams are made on."

It would seem that volition necessarily implies ideation, which defines the act to be carried out, be it one of movement, or of directed thought, affirmation, inquiry, judgment, decision, etc. Thus the waking individual brings about directed change in experience through the medium of the idea, that is, meaning-tone and/or imagery.

In the hypnotized subject, we have the same mechanism, but a far greater variety of experience is subject to change, this change being primarily determined by the meaning-tone aroused by the words which the subject hears. With a "good" subject, within the framework of his understanding and his past experience, his entire field of awareness may be altered. This may, and frequently does, include volitional activity. Probably any sort of experience can be produced, from drive, feeling, emotion, and ideation, to hallucinatory productions constructed from units of past experience ordered in experiential space.

CHAPTER 23

Conclusions

1. Time distortion can be demonstrated in the majority of subjects in whom a moderately deep trance can be produced.

2. In all probability, the subjects actually have the experiences they allege. If this be true, then time sense can be deliberately altered to a predetermined degree by hypnotic suggestion, and subjects can have an amount of experience under these conditions that is more nearly commensurate with the subjective time involved than with the world time. This activity, while seeming to proceed at a normal or natural rate as far as the subject is concerned, actually takes place with great rapidity.

3. Retrospective falsification or elaboration does not enter into the subjects' reports, when the subjects are properly selected.

4. These experiences during distorted time are continuous.

5. Thought, under time distortion, while apparently proceeding at a normal rate from the subject's point of view, can take place with extreme rapidity relative to world time. Such thought may be superior, in certain respects, to waking thought.

6. There is some evidence that the recovery of material from the unconscious can be facilitated.

7. There is some evidence that creative thought can be facilitated.

8. There is little evidence that motor learning can be facilitated, but the problem deserves further study, especially in view of reports on "imaginary learning" in the waking state.

9. There are some findings that suggest that nonmotor learning can be facilitated.

10. We have done a good deal of work to determine whether or not mathematical mental activity can be facilitated and, to date, the answer is that it cannot. The sort of hallucinatory activity that we see in time distortion in hypnosis is built up from units of past experience, made available by association. The solving of simple mathematical and coding problems probably involves some other factor that cannot operate in distorted time.

11. Only those activities which can be constructed from elements of past experience or new combinations thereof, can proceed, in distorted time, at an increased rate relative to world time. The solving of mathematical problems obviously does not fall into this category, for the answer is not to be found in the subject's past experience.

12. These experiments suggest that it is possible, by means of time distortion in hypnosis, for a subject to experience a stipulated number of events in a "clock time" interval of the experimenter's choosing. This can be rigidly controlled. Thus, in a 5-second interval by the clock, a subject can be made to experience 10 events, similar in nature and of equal seeming duration. Then, in another 5-second interval by the clock, he can be made to experience 1,000 events similar to the previous 10. This means that *experience* per se can be *isolated* and treated in terms of countable events. In other words, the quantitation of experience would seem to be possible. Whether or not any correlation can be found between the "magnitude" of two such groups of countable events (based on the number of events) and physiological or other psychological processes, remains to be seen.

PART II

The Clinical and Therapeutic Applications of Time Distortion

Milton H. Erickson, M.D.

PHOENIX, ARIZONA

The Clinical and Therapeutic
Applications of Time
Distortion

INTRODUCTION

The discovery or development of a new concept in science poses difficult questions concerning its definition and its eventual significances and applications. In the experimental work constituting the major part of this book, the term "Time Distortion" has been used as offering a reasonably concise way of expressing a methodology for a study of time itself as one of the essential elements in the experience of human living. To so emphasize time as an integral part of human experience may be considered trite, but it is not trite to recognize time as an element fully as worthy of investigation as any other factor in human living. Yet such investigative studies have been seriously neglected. From recognition of this oversight and long interest in the experiential significance of time came the senior author's impetus for the foregoing experimental studies.

In sharing with him a small part of the experimental studies, this writer became interested in the question of the clinical and therapeutic applications of the experimental findings. The publication of the first experimental study (3) suggested definite possibilities of new and better understandings of psychological functionings and, consequently, of different and more searching procedures and methodologies in dealing with psychological problems. Subsequent experimental studies and tentative applications of the findings to clinical work confirmed that first impression. In the second experimental study (4), these impressions have been discussed in the form of a general summary as follows:

Foremost to this writer are the implications of time dis⁺ortion in the field of psychotherapy. Certainly no one questions the importance of the subjective experiential life of the individual, nor the present unsatisfactory, laborious, time-consuming, and unscientific methods of studying it.

What constitutes a subjective reality? Of what seemingly pertinent and irrelevant elements is it comprised? In what way is it integrated into the total life of the person? What self-expressive purposes does it serve for the personality? What determines its validity? How does it differ from a memory, a dream, a fantasy and from retrospective falsification? In what way is it distorted by present methods of concurrent or retrospective reporting, and how much time does it require? All of these considerations are touched upon either directly or indirectly in this study and each of them constitutes a significant problem in psychotherapy, to say nothing of psychology in general.

The girl who, in an allotted 10 seconds, subjectively experienced in voluminous detail a 30-minute automobile ride upon which a report could be made with "stills" of the scenes, demonstrated a challenging possibility of a new approach to the exploration of the experiential past of the individual.

The subject who found it impossible to demonstrate in the waking state her experiential behavior in picking flowers because it was under a "different" time limit and work limit, and yet, weeks later in a trance state was able to demonstrate in actual accord with the previous findings, discloses the possibility of controlled studies of subjective realities.

Delusions and hallucinations have long constituted intriguing problems. They are subjective realities accepted by the person as objective realities. Yet, one of our experimental subjects experienced dragging a basket of apples with such vividness that he expected the experimenter to note his forced respirations, which, similar to the basket, were only subjectively real. Nevertheless, he recognized the total experience as entirely subjective but did so without it losing the experiential feeling of its objective reality. Experimental studies patterned from this and the other similar findings above might lead to a better understanding of pathological delusions and hallucinations.

Theories of learning and memory are constantly in need of revision with each new development in experimental studies in those fields. In this regard, the findings on the subject who, in an allotted 10 seconds, took a long walk and developed a conditioned response reaction by being "jolted" by an interjected sound signal, pose definite problems for research on learning, memory, and conditioning.

Similar is the instance of the violinist who, in allotted 10-second periods, subjectively experienced playing various compositions with practice effects as attested by a competent critic. Subsequent to this study, she made use of her "special personal time" to experience subjectively practicing a difficult long-forgotten composition, and then played it successfully in reality from memory without having seen the written music for years.

In this same connection, one may speculate upon the role of motor functioning in mental learning since this violinist subjectively experienced the total process of playing the violin, studying the written music, and memorizing it, while lying supine and inactive, and yet demonstrated the actual effects of reality practice.

A tempting experimental study based on these findings would be the exhibition of a form board to naive subjects and having them in special personal time, at an hallucinatory level, practice assembling it. The findings of this study warrant the assumption that, even as motor activity facilitates learning in every day reality, subjective motor activity, as contrasted to objective, is an effective aid to memory and learning.

Another interesting, actually significant finding bears upon the validity of the experiential realities to the subjects, negates assumptions of retrospective falsification, and serves to confirm the findings of various competent experimenters that hypnosis cannot be used to induce anti-social behavior. This was the discovery, in several instances, that suggested hallucinatory activities were unexpectedly regarded as objectionable by the subjects. The reactions were essentially the same in all cases and can be illustrated by the following example.

The subject was instructed to experience herself in the role of a psychologist counseling a client relative to a problem involving epilepsy. Although willing to serve as a counselor, the experiential reality of the situation was so great that she could not tolerate the task of dealing with the problem because she felt that epilepsy was beyond the rightful scope of a psychologist and that any counseling she might offer would be unethical. Accordingly, she referred her hallucinatory client to a medical man and developed intense resentment and hostility toward the experimenter for calling upon her to violate, even at a subjective level, her personal code of ethics.

While much could be said about the implications of time distortion and the experimental findings reported here in relation to concepts of gestalt psychology, the molar psychology of Tolman, Hull's modern behaviorism and Freudian psychology, this will be left to the special interests of the reader. Time and its relationships constitutes a significant element in all psychological functioning no matter from what school of thought it is viewed. Hence, any study dealing with the element of time itself in psychological functioning must necessarily have important bearing upon every school of thought, and this concept of time distortion offers a new approach to many psychological problems.

A final item of special interest to this writer centers around the problem so pertinent in research in clinical psychology and psychotherapy, namely, the problem of how to create for a subject or a patient a situation in which to respond with valid subjective reality. Certainly, this study indicates the possibility of much more rigorous controlled research with time as aid rather than as barrier.

Since the publication of the above, opportunities have arisen from time to time to utilize or to adapt various experimental findings in clinical and therapeutic work. However, it must be noted that experimental studies and clinical work belong to different categories of endeavor. In the former, rigorous controls must be exercised and the object is the determination of possibilities and probabilities. In clinical work, the welfare of the patient transcends all other matters, and controls and scientific exactitudes of procedure must give way to the experiential needs of the patient in the therapeutic situation. Another type of measure of validity, different from the controlled scientific methodology of experimental procedure, holds in clinical work. Such a measure is constituted by the thera-

peutic results that can be definitely related to the procedure employed
and which are understandably derived from it.

GENERAL CONSIDERATIONS OF CLINICAL APPLICATIONS

Since the clinical situation of psychotherapy is not a Procrustean bed,
utilization of experimental findings and concepts must necessarily depend upon the patient's needs and desires and the attendant circumstances. It can not be a matter of furthering special interests of the
therapist. Hence, any utilization must await the opportunities and occasions presented by the patient and not represent a planned procedure
established out of context with the developing needs of the patient in
therapy.

Furthermore, the concept of time distortion does not constitute in
itself a form of psychotherapy. Rather, it offers a method by which access
can be gained to the experiential life of the patient. Any therapy resulting derives from a separate process of reordering the significances and
values of the patient's experiential subjective and objective realities.

The following case reports are those of patients who presented an opportunity to investigate the applicability of time distortion to psychotherapeutic problems. These reports are presented relatively briefly and
emphasis is placed upon the salient points. No effort has been made to
elaborate extensively upon the dynamics of the individual case, since
the purpose of the reports is to demonstrate as clearly as possible the
problem, the situation and the circumstances which led to the utilization
of time distortion, and the results obtained.

PATIENT A

The first case history illustrates an unwitting and unintentional spontaneous utilization of time distortion by a patient previous to Cooper's
initial publication. It is presented because it demonstrates not only the
use of time distortion but how, in the ordinary course of psychotherapy,
an opportunity can arise for the utilization of time distortion. Needless
to say, at the time of this occurrence, this writer was at a loss to understand what had happened, but it laid the foundation for a profound
interest in Cooper's first publication four years later.

The patient, an artist in his early thirties, sought therapy primarily
for marital problems and secondarily for personality difficulties. During
therapy, despite his success in the field of portraits, landscapes and still
life painting, he felt extremely frustrated because he had not painted a
circus picture. For more than ten years, even previous to his marriage,

he had hopelessly desired to paint such a picture but had not even succeeded in making a preliminary sketch. He had not even been able to think sufficiently clearly on the subject to speculate on what figures or scenes he might wish to portray. The entire project remained a vague undefined "circus picture".

Although his other problems were clarified during months of therapy, nothing was accomplished in this regard. Even profound somnambulistic hypnotic trances, with various techniques, elicited only the explanation, "I'm completely blocked mentally. I can't think any further than 'circus picture'." He could not even sketch a possible composition plan of vertical and horizontal lines, his usual method of working out preliminary sketches.

Since the patient wished further therapy in this connection, a deep trance was induced and he was given the following post-hypnotic suggestions:

1. Stretch a large canvas in the neighborhood of 24 x 40 inches. It may be larger or smaller—possibly a golden rectangle.

2. Secure a more than adequate new supply of paint tubes and pigments and set them up as if in preparation for painting.

3. Make out a daily hourly schedule for the next three months, blocking out hours that might be used for painting the circus picture (his usual procedure in planning a new painting).

He was then awakened and dismissed with an amnesia for trance events.

A few days later, with no realization of the post-hypnotic nature of his performance, he reported that he had made a time schedule for the next two months. This schedule would permit him, if he worked hard, to finish his present commitments within two weeks. Then, over the remaining period, there would be blocks of time totalling seventy hours which he would reserve absolutely for an effort to paint a circus picture. No mention was made in relation to the other post-hypnotic suggestions.

He was hypnotized deeply and instructed to fulfill his current commitments adequately. Then he was to set about this proposed project, working slowly, carefully and painstakingly as he always did, without rushing or hurrying. In so doing, the seventy allotted hours would pass with utter and incredible speed. Yet he would work satisfyingly and at a normal tempo. (The intended purpose of this instruction was to prevent him from feeling the burden of a long-continued task.)

All of this instruction was emphatically and repetitiously given to insure adequate understanding.

Two days later a highly excited telephone call was received from him, asking for an immediate interview.

His story was as follows: While completing a current picture, he ceased work to eat his lunch of sandwiches in the studio. While so doing, he decided to stretch a new canvas, thinking vaguely that he might use it for the projected picture.

This done, he picked up the remainder of his sandwich and found it inexplicably dry. Puzzled by this, he chanced to look at the stretched canvas and was utterly amazed to find a freshly completed oil painting of a circus scene. With intense curiosity he examined it carefully, feeling exceedingly pleased and satisfied with it. Suddenly he saw his signature in the corner (which he ordinarily appended ritualistically only when he had given his final approval to his work) and noted at the same time that the style of painting was his own. Immediately he had rushed to the telephone, observing on the way that the clock gave the hour as 6:00 p.m. All the more bewildered, he had telephoned, saying, "Something's happened. Can I see you right away?" To this account he added, "What happened? What happened?"

Since he had brought the picture with him, he was questioned about it. The performing dog in it was really a neighbor's; the equestrienne was his recently acquired second wife, the clown was himself, and the Ferris wheel was one his present wife had recently described in a reminiscence. Yet the painting as a circus picture was more than satisfying to him as a person and as a critical artist. (At art exhibitions in various states, critics have all been most favorable in their comments.)

He was much puzzled by his replies to the questioning and kept reiterating, "It's the circus picture I've always wanted but it's got nothing to do with any ideas I ever had about a circus picture. It's mine; it's a circus picture; it's what I want. But what happened?"

He was hypnotized and asked to explain.

"When I had the canvas stretched like you told me to, I knew I had plenty of time. So I worked on it as slowly and as carefully as I could. I painted just the way I always do—slowly. And I had trouble, too. I knew the clown's coat had to be blue and the ribbon and the Ferris wheel also. They had to be the same shade of blue but a different blue. I used different pigments for each one, and it was an awful slow job mixing those different pigment combinations to get the same shade of color. And I had trouble with the horse's mane. I wanted to work out an entirely new technique for that and I finally succeeded. (The critics also commented favorably on that item of technique.) But I didn't have to hurry because I had plenty of time. And then when I had it finished, I studied it a long time, making sure that it was all right and when I was finally sure, I signed it. Then I picked up my sandwich and woke up. I didn't remember a thing and when I saw the picture I got puzzled and scared. I even examined the studio doors—they were still locked on the inside. So I knew that I had better see you in a hurry. But it is a good picture. Be sure you help me to know that I really painted it."

While he now knows he painted it, his general understanding of the entire matter is sketchy and vague but his satisfaction is unchanged. A year later he commented on the "curious fact" that in daylight the three shades of blue are identical but that under different lighting effects they are dissimilar. From this he had "deduced" that he "must have used different pigments."

Therapy was terminated a few sessions after the completion of the picture.

Comment

Regardless of the dynamics involved, the hypnotic suggestions given, and the purposes served for the patient, one fundamental fact remains. This is, that a task conceived of as requiring, on the basis of long experience, a total of about seventy hours, was accomplished in six with no known preliminary preparation, at a totally unexpected time and in a fashion alien to established patterns of behavior and work. The parallelism between this report and many of the experimental findings reported in the first part of this book is at once obvious and pertinent.

PATIENT B

This next case report is decidedly different. It is an example of the intentional therapeutic use of time distortion as a consequence of a failure to secure results by other methods. And since therapy was the desired goal, there was no opportunity to utilize the clinical situation to demonstrate time distortion *per se*. Rather, its existence as a reality in the situation was assumed and all efforts were directed to the securing of therapeutic results as a direct outcome of its utilization.

The patient was a thirty-year-old twice-married woman who was known to have suffered from recurrent episodes of hysterical amnesia characterized by essentially complete personal disorientation. These attacks dated from two years prior to her second marriage six years ago. Since it had been a hasty war-time marriage, her second husband knew practically nothing about her past except that she was a widow with two children, and that she had recurrent "sick spells when she didn't know nothing".

She was first seen in consultation while hospitalized with amnesia. She gave the date as 1934 and described herself as a woman but could give no other information. She did not recognize her name, her husband or her children. She complained of a severe headache and her appearance and behavior corroborated this complaint.

She made, as was usual for her, a sudden spontaneous recovery after three weeks in the hospital and left hurriedly in a state of terror upon discovering where she was.

She was seen at home the next day. She was fully oriented but still frightened. She explained that many times in the past she had suddenly awakened in a hospital after being unconscious for days at a time or even weeks. However, she was uncooperative about further questioning or therapy.

She was seen again five months later. During that time there had been a number of brief amnesic periods during which she had been cared for at home by constant supervision. Now she was again amnesic and the only information that could be elicited was that she was a woman and the year was 1934. She was hospitalized and heavily sedated for a week. She then made her usual sudden spontaneous recovery but this time she was cooperative about therapy.

She was interviewed daily for the next three months from two to four hours each day. Only a scanty outline history of her present marriage could be obtained. As for her previous life experiences, she knew only that she had been widowed, but not the year, although she knew the birthdates of her children. Nothing more of apparent significance was elicited. Mention of the date 1934 was without any apparent meaning to her. She expressed doubts about the correctness of her first name. This lack of knowledge of her past was most frightening to her and every inquiry caused her intense anxiety.

Concerning her amnesic states, she regarded them as periods of un-consciousness. She described them most unsatisfactorily. Typical of her accounts is the following: "When I woke up in the hospital, the last thing I remembered was walking down the street when a truck came along." Or, it could have been going to the store or reading a newspaper.

During those first three months every possible effort was made to secure some understanding of her problem. Since she proved to be an excellent subject, every hypnotic technique known to the writer was employed to no avail. While she could be regressed in age, such regression was limited to the relatively normal happy periods of the past eight years. Indeed, every effort to reconstruct her past by whatever technique was restricted to some limited period of the recent past. Automatic writing and drawing, crystal gazing, dream activity, mirror writing, free association, random utterances (i.e., every fifth, eight or tenth word that comes to mind), depersonalization, disorientation, identification with others, dissociation techniques and other methods were futile. Yet it was obvious that she was trying to cooperate but only relatively meaningless material of the recent past was secured.

Additionally during this time, she developed frequent amnesic states of one to three days' duration. During them she always gave the date as 1934. While she could be hypnotized deeply in these states, and hypnotic phenomena elicited, these were restricted and limited in character to various aspects of the actual office situation. Thus, she did not recognize the writer but did regard him as a possibly friendly stranger. She viewed the wall calendar as "some kind of a joke" since it did not read 1934. She could hallucinate readily and would count the books in an hallucinatory book-case. She would write simple sentences upon request, but did not seem to understand what was meant when efforts were made to have her write her name, geographical location or age. Nothing that impinged upon her personal life seemed to be comprehended. However, to a colleague experienced in hypnosis, but unacquainted with her, she was obviously in a trance. She would awaken from these trances in the amnesic state.

These amnesic periods usually terminated after a night's sleep, or, if more than a day in duration, responded to heavy sedation.

On one occasion, in the writer's presence, she chanced to see through the window a Borden's milk truck and immediately she developed a three-day amnesia. Several days after her recovery, during an interview she happened to see on the writer's desk, purposely placed there, a small calendar advertising Borden's milk. Another three-day amnesia occurred. Later, she was asked to copy a weekend sales advertisement. Upon reaching the item of Borden's milk, a third three-day amnesia ensued. Still later, while discussing recipes, Borden's milk was mentioned by the writer with a similar result. Finally, she was asked what a male hog was called and what a bear slept in. She gave the correct answers. She was then asked, with careful emphasis upon the key words, "What would happen if you put a boar in a den?" Her reply was simply, "I guess the bear would eat him."

However, the amnesic states were frequent and were apparently caused by a variety of other stimuli not recognized by the writer.

Every effort was made to secure some measure by which the amnesias could be interrupted or aborted. Finally, a very simple measure was found. Since she could be regressed to a previous age within the eight-year limit, and since she always gave the date as "sometime in 1934" when amnesic, the regression technique in reverse was employed. Thus, she would be hypnotized, and, in a systematic, repetitious fashion, told, "Yes, it is 1934, and the seconds and the minutes are passing one by one, and as the seconds and the minutes pass, so do the hours, and with the passage of the hours, so do the days pass. As the days pass, so do the weeks. The weeks come and go and the months pass and 1935 is coming closer and 1934 is passing, passing. And after 1935 will come 1936, which will pass, and then it will be 1937," etc., until the current time was reached. Frequent need to utilize this technique rapidly reduced the initial period of thirty minutes to less than five in bringing her out of her amnesic state. On two occasions, when she wandered away from home and was picked up amnesic by the police, her memory was promptly restored by this technique.

A laborious futile effort was made, following this success, to regress her from 1934 to 1933 or earlier. Then an effort was made, after getting her to accept the argument that there were years antedating 1934, to induce her to forget 1934 and to experience the date as 1930, with the hope of building up from that date. This and numerous variations of the general idea failed.

After three months' failure to make recognizable progress with her, it was decided to employ time distortion.

In the guise of sharing personal satisfactions in past professional experimental work, several prolonged sessions with her were devoted to presenting the general concepts and experimental procedures of time distortion, all as something of only intellectual interest to her. In so doing, it was hoped to avoid any measures of defense against this therapeutic approach.

This was done in both the waking and the hypnotic states. When she seemed to have a good comprehension of world, solar, clock, special, experiential and allotted time, time distortion, and time distortion experiments, the suggestion was offered that she might like to engage in an experiment comparable to those that had been read and explained to her. She agreed readily and seemed to be under the impression that the project was essentially a mere continuation of the already published study.

The next day she was hypnotized deeply and instructed as follows:[1]

"You have many times taken a trip in a car and enjoyed it immensely. The car was moving very rapidly. You saw this sight, you saw that scene, you said this, you said that, all in an ordinary way. The car moved fast but you were sitting quietly, just going along. You could not stop the car, nor did you want to. The telephone poles were so many feet apart and they came along one by one and you saw them pass. You saw the fields and they passed by, large fields, small fields, and you could only wait quietly to see what would be in the next field, and to see whether the next house would be brick or frame. And all the time the car went along and you sat quietly, you saw, you thought, all in your own way, at your own speed, just as it happened, and the car just kept going. You did not need to pay attention to the car, *just to what next would happen*, a field, a house, a horse or *whatever was next*.

"However, this experiment will not be a car ride. I have just used it to explain more fully to you. I could have described going through the cooking of a dinner—peeling potatoes, washing carrots, putting on pork chops—*anything that you could have done*.

"Now I'm going to give you much more time than you need to do this experiment. I will give you twenty seconds world time. But in your special time, that twenty seconds will be just as long as you need to complete your work. It can be a minute, a day, a week, a month or even years. And you will take all the time you need.

"I will not tell you yet what your experiment or task is. As soon as you nod your head to show that you are ready, I will start the stop watch and give you the signal *now* and very rapidly I will name the task and you will start at the beginning of it, the very beginning, and go right through to the end, no matter how far away it is in time. Ready? All right, listen carefully for the click of the watch, my signal, and the name of the task. *Now—from Childhood to Now—Remember!*" (The *Now* was repeated as literally a double signal.)

Her response was a tremendous startle reaction, a gasp, a marked physical slumping in her chair and a frozen facial expression.

Twenty seconds later she was told "Stop" and was asked, "Through?" "Yes."

---

[1] These instructions are probably much too elaborate, but a first experimental therapeutic effort with a new methodology is not an occasion for economy. They are presented rather fully in order to demonstrate the effort at comprehensiveness.

"Will you tell me if I awaken you?"

"Yes."

For several hours there was a tremendous outpouring of her past traumatic memories. These were related in a most remarkable fashion. She detailed them as if they were actually in the course of happening, or as if they were items of the very recent past and, at the same time, in a dissociated fashion, she offered comments and interpolated remarks bearing upon much later events. For example, she began her account with:

> "My dress is pink. It's my birthday. I'm sitting in a high chair. I'm going to eat my cake. My daddy is going to kiss me. He falled down. That's what happened. My father died of heart failure. I was three years old. Pink dress. When Deborah (her daughter) wanted a pink birthday dress I forgot everything and I went to the hospital. I couldn't think. My head ached. . . . I'm going on a train ride. Mummie is taking me. It's fun. See the pretty trees. There's cows, too. Mummie is coughing. She's sick. Her handkerchief is all red. (Pulmonary hemorrhage.) I'm scared. My mother is so sick. And every time Elaine (her second daughter) had a nose bleed, I got sick. . . . My hands hurt—he's going to hurt me. I can't get away. . . . I'm so tired and thirsty—he keeps doing it— he's going to kill me—I wish somebody would come." (This was a long story of being tied hand and foot to a bed for three days and repeatedly raped by a man named Borden.)

Another account was that of her delivery in 1934 of her stillborn child resulting from the raping, and her vivid report of the delivery scene and her grief over it. "That's when everything in me died. I couldn't stand to remember."

Three more instances that may be cited are her first husband's infidelity and the finding of a love letter from his paramour in his effects, and her present husband's receipt of a letter from a former fiancée, with a consequent amnesia resulting for her; the suicide of one of the girls in the maternity home during her own stay there by hanging from a chandelier, and her own daughter of similar age tying crepe paper to a chandelier as a Christmas decoration; and the inexplicable death of her third child while lying in bed one night, and reading a newspaper account of a similar instance. All of these were vividly described in the present tense and then related to actual amnesic episodes.

There were many more comparable traumatic experiences recalled and discussed, all in chronological order. This required many hours before she could complete her review of her past. Various of the events could be verified, some appeared to be hysterical fantasies of a morbid character and yet later some of these were found to be true.

Her therapeutic response to this catharsis was decidedly good. However, there were several more brief amnesic episodes but each time she recovered promptly and was able to define the precipitating stimulus and to relate it to either an incompletely discussed trauma or to one that had been overlooked. In each instance the precipitating stimulus lost its effect upon her. For example, upon moving to a new location, she readily purchased her milk from the Borden truck that travelled that street.

Shortly after all this her husband deserted her. She responded by divorcing him, securing employment and supporting her children adequately. Her employers thought highly of her.

Therapy was discontinued upon her gaining employment, except for brief casual visits at long intervals.

In final appraisal, two years after termination of therapy, she was still an hysterical personality type, but well controlled, and functioning at an adequate personal, social and economic level.

Comment

What happened during that eventful twenty seconds after months of futile effort, and how it happened, can be speculated upon best in terms of the experimental findings reported in the first part of this book. That the previous work with the patient quite probably laid the foundation for the final outcome does not militate against the significance of what occurred in twenty seconds time.

Her narrative of what happened, extended over many hours, was given largely in the present tense. Yet at the same time, it was given with interpolated comments and explanations relating long past events of her life with those of the recent past. This indicates that the narrative was not a simple initial revivification of the past. Rather, it strongly suggests that in those twenty seconds she had achieved a sufficiently comprehensive recollection of her life history to be able to see it in meaningful perspective. Then, in her narrative, couched in the terms in which she had reacquired her memories, she communicated it to the writer for his understanding and at the same time achieved for herself an effective catharsis of her experiential past.

Before utilization of time distortion, therapy was a clinical failure. Twenty seconds of time distortion, whatever that may mean clinically, resulted in a therapeutic success of a known two years' duration.

PATIENT C

This case report concerns a relatively circumscribed emotional problem for which the concept of time distortion was employed as an expeditious and experimental measure.

The patient, a twenty-five-year-old student, working his way through college, was primarily interested in the field of entertainment. His voice was fair and he accompanied himself on a guitar. Because of his promise as a singer, a night club gave him regular week-end employment. Unfortunately, as the weeks went by, his performance showed no improvement and he was notified that he would be replaced at the first opportunity.

This had caused him much discouragement, anxiety and depression and he sought therapy because of his hopeless attitude.

His history disclosed nothing of immediate significance except that his studies and his regular week-day employment on a late shift, in addition to the week-end engagement, gave him practically no time for practice.

Further inquiry disclosed that his late shift was characterized by spurts of activity followed by intervals of idleness.

This fact suggested a possibility for utilizing time distortion. Accordingly, the question of hypnosis was raised with him and he dispiritedly expressed his willingness to try anything. He proved to be a good hypnotic subject and was easily trained in hypnotic phenomena.

This accomplished, he was systematically instructed, under hypnosis, in Cooper's experiments on time distortion until his understanding of the general concepts was good. The suggestion was offered that he might participate in a time distortion experiment. He was disinterested in the idea but did consent reluctantly. He preferred that attention be given to his problem.

Accordingly, on a Monday, while in a profound trance, he was given a series of post-hypnotic suggestions. These were that he was to utilize, from time to time, each night the idle periods at work to develop brief 10- to 30-second trances. During these trances, at an hallucinatory level, he would have adequate special personal time to practice extensively both his singing and his playing. Since the trances would be brief in clock time, and since his practicing would be hallucinatory in character, his fellow-workers would not note more than that he appeared momentarily self-absorbed.

He was awakened with a total amnesia for the trance instructions and given an appointment for the next Monday.

He reported excitedly at that interview, "I've got a new lease on life. Saturday was the best night I have ever had. Sunday night I did so well that the boss said that if I kept on that way, I could be sure of my job. I don't understand it because I didn't get a chance all week to practice. But Sunday I got out my tape recorder and made a new recording. Then I played it and some of my old recordings for comparison. Sunday's sounded as if I had had a lot of practice. I was amazed to find out how much I had improved. I must have unconsciously ironed out some emotional kink that was interfering."

Hypnotized, he explained that he had averaged at least three long, as well as several brief, practice sessions per night. During the long sessions he went through his repertoire and the brief sessions were used for the practice of individual selections. Each time everything seemed to proceed at a normal tempo. Additionally, he frequently made an hallucinatory tape recording which he "played back" so that he could listen to his practicing and thus note errors for correction. At no time had any of his associates seemed to notice his periodically preoccupied state. He expressed his intention of continuing with this method of practice and supplementing it with ordinary practice.

At the present time, many months later, he still has all of his jobs and his weekend stipend has been greatly increased. He has enlarged his repertoire and he practices at every opportunity in the ordinary state and in post-hypnotic trances in time distortion.

He is still unaware of his trance activities but is greatly amazed at the rapidity with which he learns new selections.

To date he has made no effort to apply this special learning in any other way. Nor has such a suggestion been offered to him since the excellent therapeutic result might possibly be jeopardized by other experimental efforts.

Comment

This case report is essentially a parallel of some of the experimental findings reported by Cooper. While the validity of this report rests upon the bare facts of the patient's statements and his continued employment at an increased stipend, there can be no question that the concept of time distortion served a significant personality purpose for the patient. Additionally, of particular note, is the fact that the patient elaborated the suggestions given him by including an hallucinatory tape recorder to further still more the hallucinatory practice sessions, and that he has continued to utilize time distortion in learning new selections.

PATIENT D

The manner in which this patient sought therapy was both challenging and baffling. Her seemingly impossible demand was met by the utilization of time distortion which resulted in amazing and surprisingly rapid therapeutic results.

She was a nineteen-year-old girl, employed in a dental office, and she suffered from a severe reaction to the sight of blood. Usually she fainted, although occasionally she became only nauseated and greatly distressed. Otherwise she was a competent and willing employee and genuinely interested in dental work. She was directly referred for therapy by her employer who expressed a hope to retain her services and at the same time a fear that her behavior of the past few months precluded any such hope.

She arrived at the office accompanied by a chaperone. She seated herself and smoothed her dress down with exaggerated modesty and was utterly brief and final in her statements. She declared that she had come for therapy, that this was to be accomplished in a single interview and that hypnosis was to be employed.

The protest that she was demanding a miracle was disregarded by her. She merely reiterated her demand.

When asked for her history, she replied, "The doctor (her employer) has already told you over the phone. All the time I've worked for him, I've fainted every time I saw blood and I hate being picked up off the floor over and over again. I'm going to lose my job and I want to work in a dental office. That's my ambition. That's all you need to know. Now, I want to be cured. I want you to hypnotize me right away and cure me." It was as if she had indicated an aching tooth and she was demanding an extraction.

A deep somnambulistic trance was induced with remarkable ease. Asked if she were ready for therapy, she shook her head negatively and asked that "things" be "changed". This cryptic request led to an inquiry about the chaperone's presence. She asked that the chaperone be dismissed "tactfully".

When this was done, she hastily and with great urgency declared, "I'm scared—I don't know why—I'm afraid to think *and I won't think.* You have got to hypnotize me some more or I'll wake up—I just can't stay asleep. Just keep me asleep and *don't let me wake up.* You have got to help me *but don't let me know about it until it's all over* and do it fast or I'll wake up and faint. *I don't want to know anything and I don't want you or anybody else to find out what's wrong.* So don't try to find out and don't let me wake up." Much of this was repeated with emphasis.

She was assured that her wishes would be met to the fullest extent. The suggestion was offered that, first of all, it might be well to have her experience, as a means of keeping her hypnotized and as a measure of giving her satisfaction, the various common phenomena of the hypnotic trance. She agreed readily as if being given a reprieve, but admonished the writer not to forget the problem of therapy afterwards.

For fifty minutes she enjoyed thoroughly experiencing a great variety of the common hypnotic phenomena. Care was exercised constantly neither to impinge upon her personal life in inducing the hypnotic manifestations nor to seek any understanding of her as a person.

She was then told, while still in the trance, that there remained a couple more phenomena which she could enjoy. One of these was related to time and would really center around a stop watch, which was exhibited to her.

With every effort to be instructive, she was reminded of the rapidity with which time passed when she was pleased, how slowly when bored, the endlessness of a few seconds' wait for an intensely regarded outcome of a matter in doubt, the rapidity with which a mere word could cause to flash through the mind the contents of a well-liked book or the events of a long, happy trip and the tremendous rapidity and momentum of thought and feelings.

Against this background, a detailed elaboration was presented of the concept of distorted, personal, special or experiential time as contrasted to clock time. Extensive discussion was also offered of the "normal tempo" of distorted or experiential time.

When she seemed to understand, the explanation was offered that this hypnotic phenomenon could be initiated for her by giving simple instructions which she could easily accept fully. These instructions would be followed by the starting signal of "Now", at which time the stopwatch would be started. Then, when the phenomenon had been completed, she would be told to stop. This explanation was repeated until she understood fully.

Then with compelling, progressive, rapid, emphatic, insistent intensity, she was told, "Begin at the beginning, go all the way through in normal experiential tempo with a tremendous rush of force, skipping nothing, including everything, and reach a full complete understanding of everything about *Blood—Now.*"

She reacted to the word "blood" by a violent start, trembled briefly, became physically rigid, and clenched her fists and jaw. She appeared to be in acute physical distress but too rigidly involved physically and mentally to break into disruptive actions.

Twenty seconds later, at the command "Stop", she relaxed, slumped in the chair and breathed hard.

Immediately she was told emphatically, "You now know, you understand, you no longer need to fear. You don't even need to remember when you are awake, but your unconscious now knows, and will continue to know and to understand correctly, and thus give to you that ease you want."

She was asked if she wished to awaken or to think things through. Her reply was, "I've done my thinking. Wake me up."

Her waking remarks were, "I'm all tired out. I feel simply washed up. Where is Miss X (the chaperone)? What's been going on—did you put me in a trance—did she see me?"

The reply was made that she had been hypnotized and given an opportunity to learn hypnotic phenomena but that Miss X had not been a witness. She asked that Miss X be summoned and some unimportant demonstration be given to show Miss X what hypnosis was.

When this had been done, she remarked, "I suppose I owe you a fee, but I don't even know why. But I am going to make you wait for it. I don't know why."

She was told to return in one month's time. She replied, "I suppose I will, but there is no reason to do so," and thereupon took her departure.

Late the next day her employer telephoned, stating, "Whatever you did, worked. She has assisted all day in comfort, handling extracted teeth, washing out bloody trays, and even picking up bloody teeth and examining them. I haven't said a word about you nor has she and I don't think it wise."

Three weeks later part of the fee was received. A week later, she came in to say, "I don't know why you want to see me. There is no reason. I've had to get another job. My boss is going into the Army. So I've got another job. It's with Dr. Y (a dentist who does extractions). I like being a dental assistant."

A few days later a telephone call was received from her. She inquired about the balance of the bill and expressed regret for having overlooked it. Asked about her work, she declared that it was wonderful and that she would place a check in the mail immediately, as, indeed, she did. Her good adjustment is known to have continued for more than a year.

Comment

To discuss this report without emphasizing the obvious is difficult. One can readily state that it demonstrates that sometimes brief psychotherapy can be remarkably effective; that the dictum that the unconscious, if therapy is to be achieved, must be always made conscious warrants serious doubt; and that the concept of time distortion lends itself in a remarkable way to clinical therapeutic work.

What the patient's problem was and the nature of its causes remain unknown, even to her conscious mind. That it was a circumscribed neurosis is a reasonable probability. Equally probable is that therapy by other methods, given more cooperation, could have led to a similar therapeutic result. However, the fact remains that, whatever her problem was and how the therapy was achieved, the concept of time distortion proved applicable and effective under adverse conditions in meeting adequately the patient's needs.

PATIENT E

The following case is reported for two reasons. It illustrates a problem comparable to the preceding case history in that, despite much previous therapy, the entire therapeutic result was determined by the handling of a single session. Secondly, the crucial situation was one in which time distortion could have been used most advantageously but was not, since it antedated Cooper's experimental work. Viewed in retrospect, however, in terms of what happened and the final result, the utilization of time distortion could easily have resolved the ominous difficulties that developed.

Two young women in their mid-twenties had been intimate friends since early childhood. Now they were roommates and engaged in the same occupation. Each had influenced the other in the choice of work. Both were members of a minority group and had grown up in a community rife with prejudice. Both encountered prejudice in their daily work. Each confided in the other and they regularly exchanged sympathy and encouragement. Their identification with each other was remarkably strong and their relationship was definitely sisterly in type. Their adjustment within their own group was good, but they were both regarded as decidedly neurotic and they themselves recognized their neurotic patterns of behavior. Each encouraged the other to seek psychotherapy but neither had the courage to do so for herself.

Their neuroses deepened and one night Kay complained that all day she had felt strange and different. Peg tried to comfort her but found her peculiarly unapproachable. The next morning Kay was even more disturbed and on the way to work her erratic behavior attracted the attention of the police. When hospitalized she manifested an acutely catatonic state.

For about a month, Peg brooded over Kay's condition, wondering obsessionally if she should "let myself go like Kay did". Her work performance failed greatly, and she spent much time staring into space.

Finally, and reluctantly, she decided to seek therapy. Four psychiatrists were consulted, two of whom stated that their schedule was too full. The other two declared that they did not have the training requisite for her problem. She was then referred to the writer. Inquiry of the other psychiatrists disclosed that they felt that she was an "incipient, if not an actual catatonic", and not amenable to therapy at the time.

Hypnotherapy was employed from the beginning, but progress was slow, uncertain and difficult. Frequently she appeared on the verge of an acute psychosis. Repeatedly during interviews, both in the waking and the trance states, she would ponder the idea of "giving up" and "letting myself go just the way Kay did".

One evening she entered the office for her usual appointment wearing a completely new outfit, including even hat, shoes and handbag. Most seriously and in a frightened manner, she declared, "I don't know what I'm doing. I can't afford these clothes. Either I'm going to improve or I'm having a last fling before they lock me up. Maybe my unconscious knows."

With this remark she closed her eyes and developed a deep hypnotic trance.

She was asked why she had purchased the new clothes. She answered, "I don't know. Either I'm going to get well or I'm going to get worse. Wake me up."

She aroused with an apparent amnesia for her trance state. Immediately she asked, "Instead of working, can't we have a little casual conversation?"

However, after a few commonplace remarks, she declared suddenly that she had just remembered that she had dreamed the previous night. This dream, she knew, was tremendously important, but she could not recall its content. Perhaps a little reflection would enable her to remember it.

After a couple of minutes of thoughtful silence, she leaped to her feet and screamed, "No, no, I won't remember any more. I won't. I won't. It's too horrible. I'm going to forget it so that I can never remember the rest of it. It's too horrible. I'd go crazy if I remembered it."

Then, speaking to herself, she proceeded to utter a whole series of auto-suggestions, patterned after the writer's technique of suggestions, to induce an amnesia. She concluded then with a self-satisfied remark, "I've just forgotten something, I don't know what it was even about, but I do know that I can't even think of what it might be. It's completely forgotten."

In a subdued, frightened way, she continued, "I know I've done something I shouldn't have done, but I don't know what it was. It was something about forgetting, but what I don't know. It was wrong, but I'm glad I did it, awfully glad. But now I will have to give up therapy because there is no hope for me, and I'm glad. Good night!"

With difficulty she was persuaded to remain at least long enough for a social visit, but she kept declaring, "It's no use."

However, she was finally induced to review superficially and disinterestedly some of the work of previous sessions, but was adamant in her refusal to permit further hypnosis.

Finally she was persuaded to allow the writer to try to find out what she had done that was wrong and which had made everything "all over" for her. She agreed reluctantly, but again stipulated that hypnosis was not to be employed.

A whole series of speculations was offered to her, among which, in random order, were included, dreaming, remembering a dream, and forgetting a dream. She listened attentively and thoughtfully but discarded every possibility named.

She then announced her intention of leaving at once and going to visit Kay, "because I'm going to do something horrible when I get to her ward."

The plea was offered that she stay a little longer to please the writer. She yielded reluctantly but began pacing the office. She smiled to herself, pirouetted, waved her arms, giggled, and now and then stared abstractedly into space. Her attention could be secured fairly readily, although only briefly.

At last, after much persuasive effort, she consented to be hypnotized but declared that she would terminate the trance and walk out of the office, never to return, if there were any hint at therapy or even investigation of her ideas.

A number of trances were induced and utilized to elicit demonstrations of the common hypnotic phenomena in an impersonal manner.

When an effort was made to induce crystal gazing, she protested that that measure had been used therapeutically with her. She was reassured by having her hallucinate a rose bush and count the roses on it.

However, any attempt at depersonalization, disorientation, or regression elicited prompt protest and threats of waking and leaving.

More than four futile hours were spent in laborious efforts to gain control of the situation. In retrospect, the concept of time distortion could have been readily and easily utilized. With the first development of her adverse reaction, there could have been made a shift from the therapeutic situation to a simple experimental situation involving distorted time. Then, in all probability, her behavior would have paralleled that of Patients B or E.

However, after this extensive effort with her, a solution of the situation was finally reached by means of a simple, fortunate stratagem.

She was told, "Since you are terminating therapy and I shall not see you again, I would like to ask a parting favor. I hope you will grant it. It is this. You entered the office wearing a new outfit and I was glad to see you. Now I would like to hypnotize you and send you out of the office to enter it again as you did earlier, so that once more I can have the pleasant feeling I had when I first saw you tonight. Will you do this?"

She agreed and a deep trance was induced. She was instructed, "Leave the office, walk up the hall a short distance, turn and then *come down the hall and enter my office in exactly the way you did upon arriving, feeling and believing as you enter that you have just arrived and give me the same initial greeting.*"

In her willingness to grant this parting favor, she was so attentive to the actual wording of the instructions that she failed to perceive their significant implications.

She obeyed the instructions exactly and thus reentered the office regressed in time to the moment of her original arrival. Thereby, an amnesia had been effected for everything that had already occurred in the office.

In this new psychological setting, it became relatively easy to guide a second course of developments.

By techniques of dissociation, depersonalization, disorientation and crystal gazing, the patient was enabled to achieve adequate insight into and understanding of both the dream and the uncooperative disturbed behavior related to it.

Thereafter, the course of therapy was favorable and rapid and it was soon terminated as successful. More than eight years have verified this judgment.

Comment

Perhaps technically this case report, like that of Patient A, may be regarded as not belonging properly to this series. However, it illustrates, and all the more clearly since it is in retrospect, how the concept of time distortion, had it been available, could have been applicable and effective in an extremely difficult therapeutic situation. In its absence, hours of futile anxiety, which certainly did not benefit the patient, had to elapse until a fortunate stratagem of psychological maneuvering met the patient's needs. Otherwise, the probable outcome would have been regrettable.

Furthermore, this case presentation illustrates the constant need, in every field of endeavor, to review the past in terms of newer understandings and, thus, to achieve a better comprehension of both the old and the new.

PATIENT F

This final case report concerns a difficult psychiatric problem in which therapeutic progress was exceedingly slow and difficult until resort was had to the utilization of time distortion.

The patient, in his mid-twenties, complained of a variety of symptoms. He suffered from overwhelming obsessional fears of homosexuality; he had frequent disabling headaches; he was extremely fearful and shy; he lived from day to day without any interests; he was both agoraphobic and claustrophobic; and he was afraid to look at women because they became hideous creatures in some inexplicable way that caused him to be afraid to look at them.

These symptoms, of more than six months' duration, had developed rapidly some eighteen months after he had completed his military service but he could not attribute them to any particular set of circumstances nor to any particular time. They had merely developed with such distressing rapidity that he was not able to remember their onset nor the order in which they appeared.

The personal history he gave disclosed little of recognizable significance nor was he at all interested in discussing it. His concern was a repetitious recounting of his present condition.

However, it was learned that his military history was creditable and that he had had active combat experience. Upon discharge from the Army, he had systematically visited numerous relatives in the East and then had come to Arizona for employment.

Shortly thereafter, his father and stepmother had moved to Arizona because of his father's health. While he did not live with them, he visited them weekly until shortly before entering therapy and he supported them willingly. His relationship with them both had always been and still was good.

His mother had died "when I was just a little boy. It was on my tenth birthday. She was awful good to us kids. There were eleven of us.

She died suddenly, I guess it was her heart. We were awful poor and it was a really tough struggle. We were glad when Dad married Mom. Things got easier then."

Further extensive questioning elicited one other item of possible significance. This was that shortly prior to the onset of his symptoms, contrary to his usual habit, he had slept poorly and had had most disturbing dreams, none of which he had remembered subsequently.

Then one morning on his way to work he saw a pretty girl, but a closer look disclosed her to have the hideous appearance of a "rotting corpse". This terrified him. Further down the street he saw another girl approaching, and, as they met, she too assumed the appearance of a "rotting corpse". Doubts of his sanity came to his mind and these were reinforced by the discovery that every female he met became transformed into a similar revolting sight. When he finally reached the large factory room where he worked with a score of other men, he felt protected and most grateful to them, but drawn to them emotionally in a "horrible sentimental way".

Thereafter journeying back and forth and working became nightmare experiences for him.

On payday he had to stand in line in a small office to receive his check from a young female clerk. He became oppressed by the small size of the room and felt hopelessly trapped. Following this, he was unable to sleep in his room unless the windows were open and the door slightly ajar, and repeatedly during the night he would awaken to see if all were well.

He sought therapy because he felt himself on the verge of insanity, with suicide the only other possible alternative.

Therapeutic interviews for many weeks yielded little more than a compulsive repetitious recounting of material already related. He was averse to hypnotherapy and insisted that if he talked long enough, he would succeed in "talking it out".

Finally, since his funds were being exhausted, he was persuaded to permit hypnosis as a possible stimulant to more rapid progress. However, he emphasized that actual therapy must be limited to the waking state. Accordingly, it was agreed that the hypnosis would be employed simply to give him access to unconscious material which could then be discussed in the waking state.

He proved to be a good subject and, after intensive training to insure a good hypnotic performance, his permission was asked for a therapeutic investigation. This was refused and he insisted anew on only waking therapy.

Accordingly, he was told that an experiment requiring ten to twenty seconds' time could be done that would undoubtedly enable him to get at the core of his difficulties. Reassured by the brevity of the time required, he consented readily.

He was systematically taught a working knowledge of time distortion in much the same fashion as has been described above.

When this had been completed, he was given the following instructions:

"With this stopwatch I will give you an allotted world time of twenty seconds. In your own special experiential time, those twenty seconds will cover hours, days, weeks, months, even years of your experiential life. When I say 'Now', you will begin the experiment. When I say 'Stop', you will be finished. During that twenty seconds of world time, you will sit quietly, neither speaking nor moving, but mentally, in your unconscious, you will do the experiment, taking all the experiential time you need. This you will do thoroughly, carefully. As soon as I give you the starting signal, I will name the experiment and you will do it completely. Are you ready?

"Now—Go through all the causes of your problem. *Now*.

"Stop."

Immediately he awakened, sighed deeply, wiped the perspiration from his face and stated, "It was my mother. She always told me to trust her. I was so mad when she died and I hated her."

He paused, and then went on to explain, very much as Patient B did but with much less tendency to vivify so intensely. He employed tenses in a comparable fashion and interpolated explanations similarly.

A summary of his utterances is as follows:

"I was a little boy sitting in her lap. I came home from school and I fell and bit my tongue and she told me to trust her. That was her way of comforting, I suppose, but I didn't understand. The cat scratched me (rubbing his hand). Always she said 'Trust me.' She promised me a birthday party when I grew up. I waited and waited—hundreds of days. I can feel that waiting right now. It was so long. I waited for her to tuck me in bed—she is good. I waited for her to get me a penny for candy—I waited and waited. Always she said 'Trust me.' It all happened right here in this room but I thought I was back in Pennsylvania. I had to run home from school because I played too long and I was late. And always, always,

always I heard her say, 'Always trust Mother, just trust Mother, you can always trust Mother.' She is just saying it to me over and over and over all the years.

"I have just been growing up from a little boy. Everything that happened to me that made mother say 'Trust me' has just been happening right here.

"There were so many of them. I can tell you them if I should, I don't need to because they all led to the same thing. (He was assured that other details could be given later.)

"I was ten years old that day. Mother promised me a special birthday dinner and cake. We were too poor to have those things. I wanted it so bad. She kept telling me all day, 'Trust Mother to make your cake, the best cake you will ever have in all your life.' She is going in the kitchen, she stopped, I saw her get pale. She said her arm and shoulder hurt and she went to bed and I sat and watched her die. The last thing she said was 'Trust me.' I was mad at her—she promised me and she always told me to trust her and I did and I didn't have my birthday. I hated her—I was sad, too. I didn't know how to feel and I was scared. But I forgot all that. I just remembered it here.

"And then Dad and Mom came to Arizona. I visited them regular. Then one day he told me confidentially that he had cancer and that the doctors said he had only a month left to live. (Actually the father lived nearly a year.) I was feeling bad about this. I heard him tell it to me just the way he did then. Then later Mom said, "This is the tenth birthday of our marriage," and I froze up stiff and I just now heard her say it again just like she did then. Then I was going to bed and trying to sleep but I kept waking up because I kept seeing dead bodies. I hated them. They were my mother. And every one of them kept saying 'Trust me.' And I tried to run to my Dad and climb into his lap and I wanted him to love me and comfort me and put his arms around me. And I could not find him anywhere and everywhere I looked, I saw Mother dead and saying 'Trust me.'

"And the next day everything began. The girls on the street, my crazy ideas.

"That's how my problem started. Now it's over with."

The patient was right. Therapy was complete except for a few more interviews. During these he reviewed various incidents of the past and discussed his confused thinking and emotions as a child and his consequent development of intense guilt reactions.

A year has passed. He is engaged to be married, and is happy and well adjusted.

Comment

One can only speculate on how long a time therapy by other methods would have required. Equally well one can wonder how time distortion, in twenty seconds, could effect a removal of such massive repressions and activate into seemingly current reality so great a wealth of experiential life.

Undoubtedly the preceding efforts at therapy and the established rapport constituted a significant and essential foundation for the therapeutic results obtained. It does not seem reasonable to this writer that, in this kind of a problem, time distortion could be used as an initial procedure. But the results do indicate that time distortion has definite clinical and therapeutic applications.

GENERAL SUMMARY

Perhaps the best way to summarize these clinical studies is to refer the reader to the conclusions at the end of the experimental section of this book. In so doing, the parallelism between the experimental findings and the clinical findings is easily recognized.

Study of the concept of time distortion by controlled experimental research led to findings of definite psychological interest and significance. The same concept was utilized independently in the totally different field of clinical and therapeutic problems. It yielded results confirmatory and supplementary of the experimental findings. The therapeutic results obtained indicate the validity of the concept of time distortion and its applicability to psychopathological problems.

There remains now the need for further and more extensive and varied study of time distortion both as an experimental psychological problem and as a useful concept applicable to clinical and therapeutic work.

PART III

Further Considerations of Time Distortion

Milton H. Erickson, M.D.
Elizabeth M. Erickson, B.A.
PHOENIX, ARIZONA

Subjective Time Condensation as Distinct from Time Expansion

Shortly after the publication of the first edition of this book, one of the authors of this new section (E.M.E.) noted a definite oversight in the development and explication of the concept of time distortion and its clinical applications. This new section is intended to correct that omission and to clarify, from a slightly different angle, the concept of time distortion and other aspects of its clinical application.

In both the experimental and the clinical sections of this book, the concept of time distortion has been developed unilaterally in relationship to the "lengthening" or "expansion" of subjective time. The converse manifestation, that is, the "shortening", "contraction", or "condensation" of subjective time has received no direct recognition or elaboration, except for brief mention in discussions to establish contrast values. However, the implications to be derived from, and the deductions warranted by, the experimental and the clinical sections of this book make apparent that time distortion as an experiential phenomenon may be either in the nature of subjective "time expansion" or its converse, "time condensation".

Though not then recognized as such, the first experimentally and clinically significant instance of hypnotic time condensation known to these writers occurred some years previous to the initial work basic to the first edition of this book.

The situation was that of a young woman trained as an hypnotic subject for the delivery of her first child. No suggestions of any sort had been given her concerning her perception of time except that she would "have a good time" and would "enjoy having her baby".

Nevertheless, spontaneously she experienced the following subjective phenomena:

1. The twenty mile automobile ride to the hospital seemed to be re-

markably rapid, despite her repeated checkings of the speedometer which always disclosed a speed within established limits.

2. The elevator ascent to the maternity floor seemed to be unduly rapid and in marked contrast to the definite slowness of subsequent rides in that elevator.

3. The delivery room preparation of the patient seemed barely to begin before it was completed.

4. Nurses seemingly dashed in and out of the hospital room, and orderlies appeared to run rapidly up and down the corridor and everybody apparently spoke with the utmost rapidity. She expressed mild wonderment at their "hurried" behavior.

5. The obstetrician "darted in and out" of the room, "hastily" checking the progress of her labor and he seemed scarcely to complete one examination before beginning the next.

6. The minute hand of the bedside clock appeared to move with the speed of a second hand, an item of bewilderment on which she commented at the time.

7. Finally, she was transferred to the delivery room cart and was "raced" down the corridor to the delivery room, where the minute hand on the wall clock was also "moving with the speed of a second hand".

8. Once in the delivery room, the transfer to the delivery table, the draping of her body, and the actual birth of the baby seemed to occur with almost bewildering rapidity.

Actually the labor lasted a total of three hours and ten minutes, and had been remarkably easy and unhurried. Detailed inquiries of the mother subsequent to delivery, supplemented by various pertinent comments she had made during labor, served to furnish an adequate account of the greatly increased subjective tempo of all the activities comprising her total experience. All of this, she explained, had "interested" her "mildly", but she had been much more interested in the arrival of her baby.

The interpretation offered at that time of her subjective experience was the simple jocular statement that she "obviously just couldn't wait for the baby".

Cooper's development of the concept of time distortion, however, makes apparent the fact that the patient, in her eagerness to achieve motherhood, spontaneously employed the process of subjective time condensation, thereby experientially hastening a desired goal.

The above case report is a strikingly illustrative example of spontaneous experiential condensation of subjective time. However, this phenomenon is one of common experience in everyday living. We all readily recognize how pleasures vanish on fleeting wings, but, to date, it has been primarily the poet who has best described time values, as witness: "Time travels in divers paces with divers persons. I'll tell you who Time ambles withal, who Time trots withal, who Time gallops withal, and who he stands still withal." (Shakespeare, "As You Like It," Act III, Sc. 2, line 328ff.)

A common general recognition is easily given to time condensation in daily living. The vacation is so much shorter than the calendar time, the happy visit of hours' duration seems to be of only a few minutes' length —indeed, too many pleasures seem to be much too brief. Unfortunately, in the very intensity of our desire to continue to enjoy, we subjectively shorten time and conversely, in our unwillingness to suffer, we subjectively lengthen time and thus, pain and distress travel on leaden feet.

These spontaneous untutored learnings from everyday experiences suggest the importance of a continued and even more extensive study of time distortion in both of its aspects of subjective expansion and condensation.

In our experience, as well as the experience of various colleagues, the ready reversal of the usual or ordinary learnings of subjective time distortions seem to be limited primarily to learnings achieved in relation to hypnosis. In this regard, a wealth of observations has been made on hypnotic subjects in both experimental and clinical situations.

To cite an example, a dental patient, who had an extensive knowledge of hypnosis and who was definitely interested in subjective time expansion, sought hypnotic training for dental purposes. The results achieved did not derive from the actual hypnotic instructions given, but were expressive of the patient's own wishes for subjective experiences. Dental anesthesia and comfort were achieved by a process of dissociation and regression by which she subjectively became a "little girl again and played all afternoon on the lawn." As for the dental experience itself, as she remembered experiencing it subjectively, she adjusted herself in the dental chair, relaxed, opened her mouth and was astonished to hear the dentist say, "And that will be all today." She surreptitiously checked her watch with his clock and then with another clock before she could believe that an hour had elapsed. Yet, at the same time she was aware of the prolonged dissociative regressive subjective experience she had had as a child for an entire afternoon.

Thus, within the framework of a single total experience, both subjective time expansion and time condensation were achieved to further entirely separate but simultaneous experiences, that is, simultaneous as nearly as the writers can judge.

Another subject, untrained in time distortion, was employed repeatedly to demonstrate hypnotic phenomena at the close of an hour long lecture. After the first few occasions, the subject developed a trance state at the beginning of the lecture which persisted until the demonstration was concluded. By chance it was discovered that thereafter the subject inevitably misjudged the lapse of time by approximately the duration of the lecture. After repeated observation of this manifestation, inquiry elicited the significant explanation from the subject, "Oh, I just stopped the clock. I didn't want to wait all that time while you lectured." By this she meant that she did not wish to experience the long wait for the close of the lecture. Instead, she had arrested subjectively the passage of time and thereby reduced it to a momentary duration. Or, as she expressed it in her own words, "You see, that way, you start the lecture, I go into a trance and stop the clock and right away the lecture is over and it is time for the demonstration. That way I don't have to wait." In other words, she had subjectively arrested the passage of time and thereby had reduced the duration of the lecture to a seeming moment.

That report is but one of many similar accounts that could be cited. One of us (M.H.E.) has repeatedly encountered over a period of years, while assisting in conducting post-graduate seminars on hypnosis, volunteer subjects, themselves physicians, dentists or psychologists, who have spontaneously developed time condensation. Furthermore, they have done this without previous training in hypnosis or in time distortion.

Usually the situation in which this manifestation developed was one wherein the teaching needs of the lecture period required the repeated withdrawal of the instructor's attention from the volunteer subject.

One such subject, in a post-trance review of his hypnotic activities in an effort to develop a more adequate understanding of hypnotic phenomena, inquired at length about the nature and genesis of his apparently altered visual perception of the lecture room clock. He explained that, during his trance state, he had been distracted and fascinated by his discovery of a repeated sporadic movement of the minute hand of that clock. This hand, he explained, did not consistently move slowly and regularly. Some of the time it did; specifically, in those periods during which the instructor kept him busy at various tasks. When left to his own devices by the instructor's attention directed to the classroom, he noted that the minute hand "would stand still for a while, then jerk ahead for maybe five minutes, pause, and then perhaps jerk ahead for another fifteen minutes. Once it just slid around a full thirty minutes in about three seconds' time. That was when you were busy using the other subject (a second volunteer). It annoyed me when you kept demanding my attention when I wanted to watch that clock." Inquiry disclosed that his awareness of the passage of time had greatly decreased. In other words, he, too, had "stopped the clock".

Another example of the experiential values of time condensation relates to the experience of a dentist who employed hypnosis extensively in his practice. Unfortunately, in the individuality of his personal technique in maintaining a trance state, he conditioned his patients to a continuing succession of verbalizations. Even more unfortunately, as he became absorbed in the intricacies of his work on the patient, he would find himself unable to verbalize. The result was that his patients would arouse from the trance state to the mutual distress of both dentist and patient. One of the writers (E.M.E.), on the basis of her own personal experience, suggested that he employ time condensation by teaching it to his patients so that they might abbreviate the time between his verbalizations and thus become unaware of his silences. The results for that dentist were excellent.

Two further instances of the clinical use of time condensation in the therapy of individual patients can be cited. The first of these concerns the report by one of us (M.H.E.) given before the Arkansas Medical Society in May 1958 on "Hypnosis in Painful Terminal Illness" and accepted for publication in 1959 by *The American Journal of Clinical Hypnosis.*

In this report an account is given of the teaching of time condensation, in association with other psychological measures, to a professional man in the last stages of painful terminal carcinomatous disease. The clinical results obtained in this patient definitely indicated a highly significant relief of the patient's distress, a part of which was directly attributable to time condensation. Particularly for this patient did time condensation appear to preclude variously a subjective awareness, memory and anticipation of pain. The usefulness in this one case suggests the possibility of its utilization as a clinical measure of reducing subjective awareness of physical distress and pain.

As a concluding illustration of time distortion involving both subjective time condensation and time expansion in a complementary relationship, a clinical history from the practice of one of us (M.H.E.) is cited. In this report, an account is given of the experimental-clinical therapeutic procedure employed in the alleviation of a symptomatic manifestation.

The patient, a fifty year old socialite, was referred by her family physician for hypnotherapy. For many years she had suffered a yearly average of forty-five severe incapacitating migrainous headaches for which there had been found no organic basis. She had often been hospitalized for these attacks because of severe dehydration and uncontrollable vomiting. The attacks lasted from not less than three hours to as long as three weeks.

Although the patient was desirous of therapy, she was incomprehensibly demanding, dictatorial and actually uncooperative as far as psychotherapeutic exploration was concerned. She wanted all therapy to be accomplished, very definitely so, within four visits at intervals of two weeks.

Hypnosis and any hypnotic procedures considered valuable by the therapist were to be employed with the exception of any psychological investigative procedures.

The entire situation was to be so handled that she was not to have any seriously incapacitating attacks, that is, attacks of over three hours duration, in the six weeks period of her therapy.

However, it was also her demand that, since she had had these headaches for many years with great regularity, she wanted them to continue but in such fashion that they would serve to meet her "hidden personality needs" but without interfering with her as a functioning personality. (The patient was intelligent, college-bred, well-informed, happily married and a devoted grandmother.) She suggested that the character of the headaches might be changed but not the frequency. However, this was but a suggestion, she declared, and she was content to rest this responsibility upon the therapist.

In reply to her, the demand was made that the therapist required as a special consideration that she report yearly to him as a form of insurance of her therapy. After careful thought, she agreed to do so for two years providing no fee was charged, but thereafter, the therapist would secure any information from her family physician.

Despite her attitude toward therapy in directing it, restricting procedures and establishing limits, she was readily accepted as a patient, since she presented an excellent opportunity for a combined experimental and clinical approach. When informed of this type of acceptance, she agreed readily.

The actual approach to her problem, in addition to being oriented to her demands, was based upon a combined experimental-clinical procedure utilizing in sequence subjectively condensed and expanded experiential time, employing the one to enhance the other.

She proved to be an excellent subject, developing a profound somnambulistic trance within ten minutes.

The first instruction given to her was that she was to accept no suggestion that was contrary to her wishes and to resist effectively any attempt to violate any of her instructions. Next she was told to execute fully all of those instructions given her in actual accord with her expressed desires. In this manner, her full responsive acquiescence was secured in relationship to both her resistances and her actual cooperation with possible therapeutic gains.

The therapeutic plan devised for her was relatively simple. The first procedure after the induction of a deep trance was to instruct her fully in the concepts of time expansion and time condensation. Then she was told that she was, without fail, to have a relatively severe migraine attack of not more than three hours duration sometime within the next week. The severity of this attack and its termination within three hours was imperative to adequate therapeutic results.

The following week, she was to have another and even more severe attack. It would differ, however, from the headache of the preceding week in that, while it would last in subjective or experiential time slightly more than three hours, it would last in solar time as measured by a stopwatch not more than five minutes.

Both of these headaches were to develop with marked suddenness, and she was to go to bed immediately and await their termination.

The patient was then awakened with an amnesia for her trance experiences and informed that she was to return in two weeks time. Meanwhile, she was not to be disturbed or distressed by any headaches she might have.

When the patient was seen two weeks later, she developed a trance readily upon entering the office. She reported that she had obeyed instructions fully, and had experienced two headaches. The first persisted two hours and fifty minutes, and the second almost five minutes. Nevertheless the second headache seemed to be much longer that the first and she had disbelieved her stopwatch until she had checked the actual clock time.

The first headache had developed at 10 a.m. and had terminated at ten minutes to one o'clock. The other had begun sharply at ten o'clock and she had seized her stopwatch for some unknown reason and had proceded to lie down on her bed. After what had seemed to be many hours, the headache had terminated as suddenly as it had begun. Her stopwatch gave the duration as exactly four minutes and fifty-five seconds. She felt this to be an error since she was certain that the time must be some-where near mid-afternoon. However, checking with the clocks in the house corrected this misapprehension.

With this account completed, the next procedure was to outline the course of her therapy for the next two weeks. To insure her full coopera-tion instead of her wary acquiescence, she was instructed that she was first to scrutinize them carefully for their legitimacy and then to answer fully a number of questions.

In this way she was led into affirming that ten o'clock in the morning was a "good time to have a headache"; that Monday morning was the preferable day, but that any day of the week could be suitable if other matters so indicated; that on occasion, it might be feasible to have head-aches on successive days and thus "to meet personality needs" for a two weeks period instead of "meeting them" on a weekly basis of one head-ache per week. It was also agreed that she would have to consider the feasibility of having a "spontaneous unplanned" headache at rare in-tervals throughout the year. These however would probably be less than three solar hours in length.

To all of this the patient agreed.

Thereupon she was instructed to have headaches of less than five minutes each beginning at ten o'clock on the next two Monday mornings.

Again she was awakened with an amnesia and dismissed.

Upon her next visit, the patient demanded an explanation of the events of the preceding two weeks. She explained that she had had two social engagements which she had cancelled because of a premonition of a headache. In both instances her premonition had been correct. Both headaches were remarkable in her experience. Both were so severe that she had become disoriented in time. Both made her feel that several hours had passed in agonizing pain but that a stopwatch she had felt impelled to take to bed with her disclosed the headaches to be only a couple of minutes in duration.

She was answered by the statement that she was undergoing a com-bined experimental-clinical hypnotherapy that was developing ade-quately and that no further explanation could be offered as yet. She ac-cepted this statement after some brief thought and then developed of her own accord a deep trance state.

Immediately she was given adequate commendation for the excellence of her cooperation, but no further explanation was offered and no in-quiries were made of her.

Further therapeutic work centered around teaching her a more adequate appreciation of subjective time values. This was done by having her, still in the trance state, determine with a stopwatch, the actual length of time that she could hold her breath. In this way it became possible to give her an effective subjective appreciation of the unendurable length of sixty seconds, to say nothing of ninety seconds.

Against this background of stopwatch experience, she was given hypnotic suggestions to the effect that, henceforth, whenever her "personality needs" so indicated, she could develop a headache. This headache could develop at any convenient time on any convenient day, and would last a "long, long sixty whole seconds" or even an "unendurably long, painfully long, ninety seconds". It would quite probably be excruciatingly painful.

When it was certain that the patient understood her instructions, she was dismissed.

She returned in two weeks to declare it was her last visit, since she expected therapy to be concluded. Thereupon she developed a profound somnambulistic trance.

She was immediately told that the therapist wished to review with her the proceedings of the previous interviews and the resulting events. She replied, "That is all so unnecessary. I remember perfectly everything in my unconscious mind. I understand and I approve and I will cooperate fully. Is there anything new you wish to tell me?"

She was reminded that it was possible that on rare occasions she might develop an "unexpected, unplanned, completely spontaneous headache."

She replied that she remembered and that if there were nothing more to be done, she wished to terminate the interview without delay. Upon the therapist's assent, she roused from the trance, thanked the therapist, stated that a check would be sent in three months' time, at which time she would send also a preliminary report.

The reports received in the next two years and from her physician since then have all disclosed that the patient benefited extensively. She has on the average about three "unexpected headaches" a year, lasting from two to four hours. At no time has she required hospitalization, as had been the case previously.

However, once a week, with ritualistic care, usually at ten o'clock on a Monday morning, she enters her bedroom, lies down on the bed, and has a headache which she describes as "lasting for hours but the stopwatch always shows it only lasts from fifty to eighty seconds. It just seems for hours. And then I'm all over every bit of it for another week. Sometimes I even have those headaches on two successive days and then I'm free for two weeks. Sometimes I even forget to have one and nothing happens."

Case Summary and General Comment

This last case history illustrates a number of important considerations. It demonstrates effectively both the value of the experimental psychological approach in psychotherapy as contrasted to traditional methods and the efficacy of an alleviation of a symptomatic manifestation when adequate allowance and provision is made for the unknown personality structure and its resistances to therapy. Also, it discloses clinical and experimental possibilities in the varied utilization of two distinct aspects of subjective time distortion.

However, of greater significance for the purposes of this book, this case history in conjunction with the material preceding it demonstrates the importance experimentally, clinically and experientially of subjective time distortion whether as time expansion or as time condensation.

References

1. BARNETT, L. The Universe and Dr. Einstein. New York: Sloan, 1950.
2. BRUNSE, A. J. Personal communication.
3. COOPER, L. F. Time distortion in hypnosis: I. Bull., Georgetown Univ. Med. Center, 1948, 1, 214–221.
4. COOPER, L. F. AND ERICKSON, M. H. Time distortion in hypnosis: II. Bull., Georgetown Univ. Med. Center, 1950, 4, 50–68.
5. COOPER, L. F. AND RODGIN, D. W. Time distortion in hypnosis and nonmotor iearning. Science, 1952, 115, 500–502.
6. COOPER, L. F. AND TUTHILL, C. H. Time distortion in hypnosis and motor learning. J. Psychol., 1952, 34, 67–76.
7. COOPER, L. F. Time distortion in hypnosis, with a semantic interpretation of the mechanism of certain hypnotically induced phenomena. J. Psychol., 1952, 34, 257–284.
8. Suggested by P. F. Cooper, Jr.
9. ERICKSON, M. H. Development of apparent unconsciousness during hypnotic reliving of traumatic experience. Arch. Neurol. & Psychiat., Dec. 1937, 38, 1282–1288.
10. INGLIS, N. R. Personal communication.
11. JACOBSON, E. Electrophysiology of mental activities. Am. J. Psychol., 1932, 44, 677–694.
12. LOVATT, W. F. Hypnosis and Suggestion. Rider and Co., London.
13. PERRY, H. M. The relative efficiency of actual and "imaginary" practice in five selected tasks. Arch. Psychol., 1939, 34, 1–76.
14. RHINE, J. B. Interview.
15. ROSEN, HAROLD. Personal communication.
16. RUBIN-RABSON, G. Studies in the psychology of memorizing piano music: VI. A comparison of two forms of mental rehearsal and keyboard overlearning. J. Educ. Psychol., 1941, 32, 593–602.
17. SAWYER, W. W. Mathematician's Delight. Middlesex, England: Penguin Books, 1943.
18. SNOW, H. L. Personal communication.
19. VANDELL, R. A., DAVIS, R. A. AND CLUGSTON, H. A. The function of mental practice in the acquisition of motor skills. J. Gen. Psychol., 1943, 29, 243–250.
20. WELCH, L. The space and time of induced hypnotic dreams. J. Psychol., 1935–6, 1, 171–178.

Index